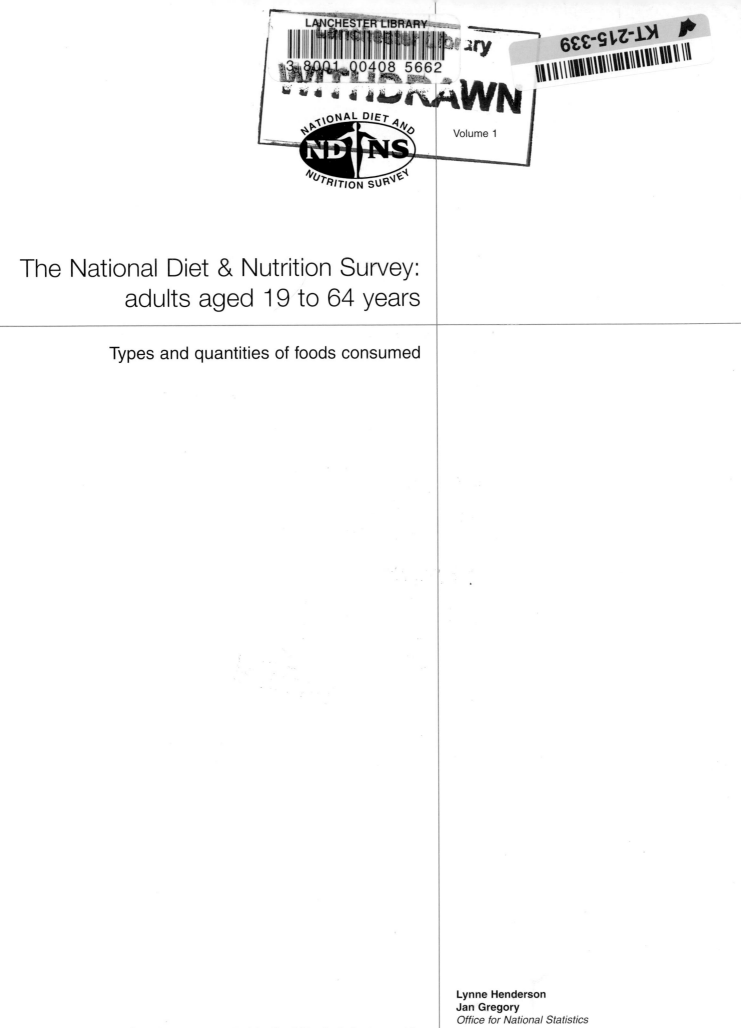

NATIONAL DIET AND NUTRITION SURVEY
ND NS

Volume 1

The National Diet & Nutrition Survey: adults aged 19 to 64 years

Types and quantities of foods consumed

Lynne Henderson
Jan Gregory
Office for National Statistics

with **Gillian Swan**
Food Standards Agency

A survey carried out in Great Britain on behalf of the Food Standards Agency and the Departments of Health by the Social Survey Division of the Office for National Statistics and Medical Research Council Human Nutrition Research

ISBN 0 11 621566 6

This report has been produced by the Social
Survey Division of the Office for National
Statistics in accordance with the Official
Statistics Code of Practice.

Contact points

For enquiries about this publication, contact
Lynne Henderson
Tel: **020 7533 5385**
E-mail: **lynne.henderson@ons.gov.uk**

Coventry University

To order this publication, call TSO
on **0870 600 5522**. See also back cover.

For general enquiries, contact the National Statistics
Public Enquiry Service on **0845 601 3034**
(minicom: 01633 812399)
E-mail: **info@statistics.gov.uk**
Fax: 01633 652747
Letters: Room D115, Government Buildings,
Cardiff Road, Newport NP10 8XG

You can also find National Statistics on the Internet
at **www.statistics.gov.uk**

About the Office for National Statistics
The Office for National Statistics (ONS) is the government
agency responsible for compiling, analysing and disseminating
many of the United Kingdom's economic. social and demographic
statistics, including the retail prices index, trade figures and labour
market data, as well as the periodic census of the population and
health statistics. The Director of ONS is also the National
Statistician and the Registrar General for England and Wales, and
the agency that administers the registration of births, marriages
and deaths there.

Contents

Foreword

This survey, of a national sample of adults aged 19 to 64 years, is one of a programme of national surveys with the aim of gathering information about the dietary habits and nutritional status of the British population. The results of the survey will be used to develop nutrition policy and to contribute to the evidence base for Government advice on healthy eating.

This report, covering foods consumed, is the first in a series to be published on the findings of this survey. Further reports covering nutrient intakes and nutritional status will be published in 2003.

The work described in this series of reports results from a successful collaboration between the Food Standards Agency and the Department of Health, which jointly funded the collection of the survey data, with the Office for National Statistics and the Medical Research Council Resource Centre Human Nutrition Research.

We warmly welcome this first report of the latest survey in the National Diet and Nutrition Survey programme and express our thanks to all the respondents who took part.

Sir John Krebs
Chairman

Food Standards Agency

Hazel Blears
Minister for Public Health

Department of Health

Authors' acknowledgements

We would like to thank everyone who contributed to the survey and the production of this report:

- the respondents without whose co-operation the survey would not have been possible;

- the interviewers of Social Survey Division of ONS (SSD) who recruited the respondents and carried out all the fieldwork stages of the survey;

- colleagues in Social Survey Division of ONS in the Sampling Implementation Unit, Field Branch, Business Solutions, Methodology Unit and Project Support Branch; in particular, Ann Whitby, Michaela Pink, Karen Irving, Caroline Ojemuyiwa, Michael Staley, Glenn Edy, Andrew Tollington, Dave Elliot, Jeremy Barton, Tracie Goodfellow and Jacqueline Hoare;

- the ONS nutritionists, namely Debbie Hartwell, Michaela Davies, Sui Yip, Laura Hopkins, Jessica Ive, Sarah Oyston, Claire Jaggers and Robert Anderson;

- the ONS editors, namely Angela Harris, Carole Austen, Mike Donovan, Nina Hall, Sue Heneghan, Sarah Kelly, Dave Philpot, Colin Wakeley, Carol Willis and Heather Yates;

- staff of the Medical Research Council Human Nutrition Research (HNR), particularly Steve Austin, Dr Chris Bates, Dr Andy Coward, Dr Jayne Perks and Dr Ann Prentice;

- Dr Maureen Birch, the survey doctor, for her input into the design, conduct and interpretation of the survey, in particular for her negotiations with NHS Local Research Ethics Committees;

- the phlebotomists and local laboratory personnel who were recruited by HNR to take the blood samples, and process and store the blood specimens;

- Professor Elaine Gunter, Chief, National Health and Nutrition Examination Survey (NHANES) Laboratory, Centres for Disease Control and Prevention, Atlanta, USA, for an independent review of the methodology for the blood sample collection and laboratory analyses;

- Professor Angus Walls for his contribution to the oral health component and briefing the interviewers on the procedures for the self-tooth and amalgam-filling count;

- Professor Chris Skinner and Dr David Holmes at the University of Southampton for an independent review of response to this NDNS and an assessment of non-response bias;

- the professional staff at the Food Standards Agency and the Department of Health, in particular Jamie Blackshaw, Susan Church, Michael Day, Melanie Farron, Tom Murray, Dr John Pascoe, Dr Roger Skinner and Alette Weaver of the Food Standards Agency; Richard Bond, Tony Boucher, Ian Cooper, Dr Sheela Reddy and Robert Wenlock of the Department of Health.

Notes to the tables

Tables showing percentages

In general, percentages are shown if the base is 30 or more. Where a base number is less than 30, actual numbers are shown within square brackets.

The row or column percentages may add to 99% or 101% because of rounding and weighting.

The varying positions of the bases in the tables denote the presentation of different types of information. Where the base is at the foot of the table, the whole distribution is presented and the individual percentages add to between 99% and 101%. Where the base is given in a column, the figures refer to the proportion of respondents who had the attribute being discussed, and the complementary proportion, to add to 100%, is not shown in the table.

In tables showing cumulative percentages the row labelled 'All' is always shown as 100%. The proportion of cases falling above the upper limit of the previous band can be calculated by subtracting from 100 the proportion in the previous band. Actual maximum values are not shown in tables of cumulative percentages, since they could vary for different subgroups being considered within the same tables.

Unless shown as a separate group, or stated in the text or a footnote to a table, estimates have been calculated for the total number of respondents in the subgroup, excluding those not answering. Base numbers shown in the tables are the total number of respondents in the subgroup, including those not answering.

The total column may include cases from small subgroups not shown separately elsewhere on the tables, therefore the individual column bases may not add to the base in the total column.

Conventions

The following conventions have been used in the tables:

..	data not available
-	category not applicable; no cases
0	values less than 0.5%
[ ]	numbers inside square brackets are the actual numbers of cases, when the base is fewer than 30.

Tables showing descriptive statistics – mean, percentiles, standard deviation of the mean

These are shown in tables to an appropriate number of decimal places.

Significant differences

Differences commented on in the text are shown as being significant at the 95% or 99% confidence levels ($p<0.05$ and $p<0.01$). Throughout this volume, the terms 'significant' and 'statistically significant' are used interchangeably. Where differences are shown or described as being 'not statistically significant' or 'ns', this indicates $p>0.05$. The formulae used to test for significant differences are given in Appendix B, pages 69–73.

Where differences between subgroups are compared for a number of variables, for example differences between respondents in different age groups in their consumption of whole milk, the significance level shown ($p < 0.05$ or $p < 0.01$) applies to all comparisons, unless otherwise stated.

Standard deviations

Standard deviations for estimates of mean values are shown in the tables and have been calculated for a simple random sample design. In testing for the significant difference between two sample estimates, proportions or means, the sampling error calculated as for a simple random design was multiplied by an assumed design factor of 1.5, to allow for the complex sample design. The reader is referred to Appendix B for an account of the method of calculating true standard errors and for tables of design factors for the main variables and subgroups used throughout this volume. In general, design factors were below 1.5 and therefore there will be some differences in sample proportions and means not commented on in the text that are significantly different, at least at the $p < 0.05$ level.

Weighting

Unless otherwise stated, all proportions and means presented in the tables in the substantive chapters in this volume are taken from data weighted to compensate for the differential probabilities of selection and non-response. Base numbers are presented weighted. All base numbers are given in italics. See Appendix C for unweighted base numbers, and Appendix D of the Technical Report online for more details on the weighting: accessible at http://www.food.gov.uk/science/ (verified November 2002).

1 Background, research design and response

This volume presents the initial findings on food intake from a survey of the diet and nutrition of adults aged 19 to 64 years living in private households in Great Britain, carried out between July 2000 and June 2001. It is the first volume in a series that will cover food and nutrient intake data derived from the analyses of dietary records, and data on nutritional status from physical measurements including anthropometric data, blood pressure, physical activity and the analyses of the blood and urine samples[1]. This first part of the report describes the background to the National Diet and Nutrition Survey (NDNS) of adults aged 19 to 64 years, its main aims, research designs and methodologies and response. The main part of this report covers the quantities of foods consumed by respondents, including an analysis of the number of portions of fruit and vegetables consumed, and differences by age, sex, region and household benefit status.

The Technical Report containing the methodological chapters and appendices is available online[2]. Like previous surveys in the NDNS programme, a copy of the survey database, containing the full data set will be deposited following publication of the final summary volume with The Data Archive at the University of Essex. Independent researchers who wish to carry out their own analyses should apply to the Archive for access[3].

1.1 The National Diet and Nutrition Survey programme

The survey forms part of the National Diet and Nutrition Survey programme, which was set up jointly by the Ministry of Agriculture, Fisheries and Food[4] and the Department of Health in 1992 following the successful Dietary and Nutritional Survey of British Adults aged 16 to 64 years carried out in 1986/87 (1986/87 Adults Survey)[5]. MAFF's responsibility for the NDNS programme has now transferred to the Food Standards Agency.

The NDNS programme aims to provide comprehensive, cross-sectional information on the dietary habits and nutritional status of the population of Great Britain. The results of the surveys within the programme are used to develop nutrition policy at a national and local level, and to contribute to the evidence base for Government advice on healthy eating.

The NDNS programme is intended to:

- provide detailed quantitative information on the food and nutrient intakes, sources of nutrients and nutritional status of the population under study as a basis for Government policy;

- describe the characteristics of individuals with intakes of specific nutrients that are above and below the national average;

- provide a database to enable the calculation of likely dietary intakes of natural toxicants, contaminants, additives and other food chemicals for risk assessment;

- measure blood and urine indices that give evidence of nutritional status or dietary biomarkers, and to relate these to dietary, physiological and social data;

- provide height, weight and other measurements of body size on a representative sample of individuals and examine their relationship to social, dietary, health and anthropometric data as well as data from blood analyses;

- monitor the diet of the population under study to establish the extent to which it is adequately nutritious and varied;

- monitor the extent of deviation of the diet of specified groups of the population from that recommended by independent experts as optimum for health, in order to act as a basis for policy development;

- help determine possible relationships between diet and nutritional status and risk factors in later life;

- assess physical activity levels of the population under study; and

- provide information on oral health in relation to dietary intake and nutritional status.

This cross-sectional study of adults aged 19 to 64 years is part of a planned programme of surveys covering representative samples of defined age groups of the population. The surveys of older adults, pre-school children, and young people have been published[6,7,8]. The last national survey of diet and nutrition in adults was the 1986/87 Adults Survey.

1.2 The sample design and selection

A nationally representative sample of adults aged 19 to 64 years living in private households was required. The sample was selected using a multi-stage random probability design, with postal sectors as first stage units. The sampling frame included all postal sectors within mainland Great Britain; selections were made from the small users' Postcode Address File. The frame was stratified by 1991 Census variables. A total of 152 postal sectors were selected as first stage units, with probability proportional to the number of postal delivery points, and 38 sectors were allocated to each of four fieldwork waves. The allocation took account of the need to have approximately equal numbers of households in each wave of fieldwork and for each wave to be nationally representative. From each postal sector 40 addresses were randomly selected[9].

Eligibility was defined as being aged between 19 and 64 and not pregnant or breastfeeding at the time of the doorstep sift[10]. Where there was more than one adult between the ages of 19 and 64 years living in the same household, only one was selected at random to take part in the survey[11]. A more detailed account of the sample design is given in Appendix D of the Technical Report[2]. In

keeping with the Social Survey Division of ONS (SSD) normal fieldwork procedures, a letter was sent to each household in the sample in advance of the interviewer calling, telling them briefly about the survey (*see* Appendix A of the Technical Report[2]).

As in previous surveys in the NDNS series, fieldwork covered a 12-month period, to cover any seasonality in eating behaviour and in the nutrient content of foods; for example, full fat milk. The 12-month fieldwork period was divided into four fieldwork waves, each of three months duration[12]. The fieldwork waves were:

Wave 1: July to September 2000

Wave 2: October to December 2000

Wave 3: January to March 2001

Wave 4: April to June 2001

Feasibility work carried out between September and December 1999 by the SSD and the Medical Research Council Human Nutrition Research (HNR) tested all the components of the survey and made recommendations for revisions for the mainstage. For a subgroup of the feasibility study sample, the validity of the dietary recording methodology was tested using the doubly labelled water methodology to compare energy expenditure against reported energy intake. Further details of the design and results of the feasibility study are summarised in Appendix C of the Technical Report[2].

Ethics approval was gained for the feasibility and mainstage survey from a Multi-centre Research Ethics Committee (MREC), and National Health Service Local Research Ethics Committees covering each of the 152 sampled areas (*see* Appendix N of the Technical Report[2]).

1.3 The components of the survey

The survey design included: an interview to provide information about the socio-demographic circumstances of the respondent and their household, medication, and eating and drinking habits; a weighed dietary record of all food and drink consumed over seven consecutive days; a record of bowel movements for the same seven days; a record of physical activity over the same seven days; physical measurements of the respondent (height, weight, waist and hip circumferences); blood pressure measurements; and a request for a sample of blood and a 24-hour urine collection. Respondents were also asked to do a self-count of the number of teeth and amalgam fillings they had, and provide a sample of tap water from the home for analysis of fluoride.

1.3.1 The dietary and post-dietary record interview

The interview comprised two parts. An initial face-to-face interview using computer-assisted personal interviewing methods (CAPI) to collect information about: the respondent's household, their usual dietary behaviour, consumption of artificial sweeteners, herbal teas and other drinks; any foods that were avoided and the reasons for doing so, including vegetarianism and dieting behaviours; the use of salt at the table and in cooking; and the use of fluoride preparations and dietary supplements. Information was also collected on: the respondent's health status; their smoking and drinking habits; socio-economic characteristics; and, for women in defined age groups, the use of the contraceptive pill, menopausal state and use of hormone replacement therapy.

There was also a short interview, using CAPI, conducted at the end of the seven dietary recording days (post-dietary record interview). Respondents were asked about any problems they experienced in keeping the diary, whether their consumption of specific foods had changed during the seven days and whether they had been unwell at all during the recording period. Respondents were also asked to complete an eating restraint questionnaire, using computer-assisted self-interviewing (CASI) or on paper. Information was also collected on prescribed medications taken during the seven days.

The interview questionnaire is reproduced in Appendix A of the Technical Report[2].

1.3.2 The dietary record

The survey used a weighed intake methodology since its main aims were to provide detailed quantitative information on the range and distribution of intakes of foods and nutrients for respondents aged 19 to 64 years in Great Britain, and to investigate relationships between nutrient intakes, physical activity levels and various nutritional status and health measures. The advantages and disadvantages of this method and the factors affecting the choice are discussed in Appendix F of the Technical Report[2].

In deciding to use a weighed intake methodology, the period over which to collect information needed to be long enough to give reliable information on usual food consumption, balanced against the likelihood of poor compliance if the recording period was lengthy. The feasibility study concluded that it was possible to collect dietary information for a seven-day period from respondents and that the quality of information would be acceptable (see Appendix C of the Technical Report[2]).

Information which would be of use to the interviewer when checking the dietary record was also collected: for example, on respondents' usual eating pattern on weekdays and at weekends; and on the types of certain common food items eaten, such as milk, bread and fat. This information was recorded on a paper form rather than in the CAPI program, so that the interviewer could use it to check diary entries during the recording period (see F7, Appendix A of the Technical Report[2]).

Respondents were asked to keep a weighed record of all food and drink they consumed, both in and out of the home, over seven consecutive days. Each respondent was issued with a set of accurately calibrated Soehnle Quanta digital food scales and two recording diaries: the 'Home Record' diary for use when it was possible for foods to be weighed, generally foods eaten in the home; and a smaller 'Eating and Drinking Away From Home' diary (the 'Eating Out' diary) for use when foods could not be weighed, generally foods eaten away from home. The respondent was also issued with a pocket-sized notebook for recording any of this information in circumstances where they were reluctant or it was inappropriate to carry the 'Eating Out' diary. The instruction and recording pages from these documents relating to the dietary information are included in Appendix A of the Technical Report[2].

The respondent, together with any other household member who might be involved in keeping the diary, for example their spouse or partner, was shown by the interviewer how to use the scales to weigh food and drinks, how to weigh and record leftovers, and how to record any food that was spilt or otherwise lost and so could not be re-weighed.

The 'Home Record' diary was the main recording and coding document. For each item consumed over the seven days a description of the item was recorded, including the brand name of the product and, where appropriate, the method of preparation. Also recorded was the weight served and the weight of any leftovers, the time food was eaten, whether it was eaten at home or elsewhere, and whether fruit and vegetables were home grown, defined as being grown in the household's own garden or allotment. The person who did the weighing, the respondent or someone else, was also recorded for each food item and, for each day, the respondent was asked to indicate whether they were 'well' or 'unwell'.

Respondents who completed a full seven-day dietary record were given a £10 gift voucher by the interviewer, as a token of appreciation. It was made clear that receiving the voucher was not dependent on co-operation with any other component of the survey, in particular, consenting to provide a blood sample.

Respondents started to record their consumption in the diaries as soon as the interviewer had explained the procedure and left the home, although the seven-day recording period started from midnight. The interviewer called back approximately 24 hours after placing the diaries in order to check that the items were being recorded correctly, to give encouragement and to re-motivate where appropriate. Everything consumed by the respondent had to be recorded, including medicines taken by mouth, vitamin and mineral supplements, and drinks of water. Respondents were encouraged to weigh everything they could, including takeaway meals brought into the home to eat. Where a served item could not be weighed, respondents were asked to record a description of the portion size, using standard household measures, or to describe the size of the item in some other way. Each separate item of food in a served portion needed to be weighed separately in order that the nutrient composition of each food item could be calculated. In addition, recipes for all home-made dishes were collected.

The amount of salt used either at the table or in cooking was not weighed, however questions on the use of salt in the cooking of the respondent's food and their use of salt at the table were asked at the dietary interview. All other sauces, pickles and dressings were recorded.

Vitamin and mineral supplements and artificial sweeteners were recorded as units consumed: for example, one Boots Vitamin C tablet 200mg, one teaspoon of Canderel Spoonful.

A large amount of detail needed to be recorded in the dietary record to enable similar foods prepared and cooked by different methods to be coded correctly, as such foods will have different nutrient compositions. Information could also be needed on cooking method, preparation and packaging as well as an exact description of the item before it could be accurately coded. Details on the recording of leftovers and spillage are given in Appendix F of the Technical Report[2]. An aide-memoire on using the scales and recording in the 'Home Diary' was left with respondents (*see* W1 and W2, Appendix A of the Technical Report[2]).

The 'Eating Out' diary was intended to be used only when it was not possible to weigh the food items. In such cases, respondents were asked to write down as much information as possible about each food item consumed, particularly the portion size and an estimate of the amount of any left over. Prices, descriptions, brand names, place of purchase, and the time and place where the food was consumed were all recorded. In certain circumstances, interviewers were allowed to purchase duplicate items which they would then weigh.

Where the respondent consumed food or drink items provided by their workplace or college, the interviewer was required to visit the workplace/college canteen to collect further information from the catering manager about, for example, cooking methods, portion sizes and types of fats used. The information was recorded on a 'catering questionnaire', which included standard questions on portion sizes and cooking methods, and had provision for recording information on specific items that the respondent had consumed (*see* Appendix A of the Technical Report[2]).

At each visit to the household, interviewers checked the diary entries with the respondent to ensure that they were complete and all the necessary detail had been recorded. Reasons for any apparent omission of meals were probed by the interviewers and noted on the diaries. If the interviewers probing uncovered food items that had been consumed but not recorded, these were added to the diary at the appropriate place. Before returning the coded diaries to ONS headquarters, interviewers were asked to make an assessment of the quality of the dietary record, in particular the extent to which they considered that the diary was an accurate reflection of the respondent's actual diet.

Interviewers were trained in and responsible for coding the food diaries so they could readily identify the level of detail needed for different food items and probe for missing detail at later visits to the household. A food code list, giving code numbers for about 3,500 items and a full description of each item, was prepared by nutritionists at the Food Standards Agency and the ONS, for use by the interviewers. As fieldwork progressed, further codes were added to the food code list for home-made recipe dishes and new products found in the dietary record. A page from the food code list is reproduced in Appendix A of the Technical Report[2].

Brand information was collected for all food items bought pre-wrapped, as some items, such as biscuits, confectionery and breakfast cereals, could not be food coded correctly unless the brand was known. Brand information was only coded for artificial sweeteners, bottled waters, herbal teas and herbal drinks, and soft drinks and fruit juices, to ensure adequate differentiation of these items. Food source codes were also allocated to each meal in order to identify food obtained and consumed outside the home. The contribution to total nutrient intake by foods from different sources could then be calculated.

After the interviewers had coded the entries in the dietary records, ONS headquarters coding and editing staff checked the documents. ONS nutritionists carried out initial checks for completeness of the dietary records, dealt with specific queries from interviewers and coding staff, and advised on and checked the quality of coding, with advice from Food Standards Agency nutritionists. They were also responsible for converting descriptions of portion sizes to weights, and checking that the appropriate codes for recipes and new products had been used. Computer checks for completeness and consistency of information were run on the dietary and questionnaire data. Following completion of these checks and calculations, the information from the dietary record was linked to the nutrient databank; nutrient intakes were thereby calculated from quantities of food consumed. This nutrient databank, which was compiled by the Food Standards Agency, holds information on 56 nutrients for each of the 6,000 food codes. Further details of the nutrient databank are provided in Appendix H of the Technical Report[2]. Each food code used was also allocated to one of 115 subsidiary food groups; these were aggregated into 57 main food groups

and further aggregated into 11 food types (*see* Appendix G of the Technical Report[2]).

1.4 Response and weighting

Table 1.1 shows response to the dietary interview and dietary record overall and by fieldwork wave. Of the 5,673 addresses[13] (*see* Chapter 2 of the Technical Report[2]) issued to the interviewers, 35% were ineligible for the survey. This high rate of ineligibility is mainly due to the exclusion of those aged under 19 years and those aged 65 or over. Just over one-third of the eligible sample, 37%, refused outright to take part in the survey. Only 2% of the eligible sample were not contacted. Overall, 61% of the eligible sample completed the dietary interview, including 47% who completed a full seven-day dietary record. Overall, 77% of those who completed the dietary interview completed a full seven-day dietary record.

While there has been a general fall in response to government social surveys over the last decade[14], the level of refusal to this NDNS was higher than expected. Steps were taken at an early stage to improve response, and included reissuing non-productive cases[15], developing the interviewer training to address further response issues, providing general guidance on approaching and explaining the survey to respondents, and increased support to the interviewers and their managers. This met with some success, so that in Wave 4 a higher proportion of the eligible sample, 67%, completed the dietary interview compared with previous waves, 56% to 60%. Those who completed the dietary record had a similar demographic profile, by sex, age and social class of the Household Reference Person as those who completed the dietary interview. (*see* also Chapter 2 of the Technical Report[2]).

The potential for bias in any dataset increases as the level of non-response increases. This is because there is an increased risk that little or no information will be collected on particular subgroups within the study population. An independent evaluation of the potential impact of non-response bias was undertaken by the University of Southampton[16]. The authors concluded that there was no evidence to suggest serious non-response bias, although this should be interpreted with caution as bias estimates were based upon assumptions about the total refusals and non-contacts for whom there was very little information. The authors recommended population-based weighting by sex, age and region. Indeed, without weighting for the differential response effect, estimates for different groups would be biased estimates because, in particular, they under-represent men and the youngest age group. To correct for this, the data presented in this volume and the other volumes of this survey have been weighted using a combined weight, based on differential sampling probabilities and differential non-response. Bases in tables are weighted bases scaled back to the number of cases in the responding and diary samples. Unweighted bases are given in Appendix C on page 74. Further details of the weighting procedures are given in Appendix D of the Technical Report[2].

In summary, the estimates presented in this report result from weighting the data as effectively as possible using the available information. However, results should be interpreted with caution, particularly where the sample sizes are low. The reader should note that the sample size in Scotland is particularly low and therefore standard errors may be large (*see* Appendix B, pages 69–73, for further details on standard errors).

(Table 1.1)

References and endnotes

1   The other volumes in this series will cover:

(i)   Macronutrient intakes (energy, protein, carbohydrates, fats & fatty acids and alcohol), to be published in early 2003;

(ii)   Micronutrient intakes (vitamins and minerals, including analysis of urinary analytes), to be published in spring 2003;

(iii)   Nutritional status (blood pressure, anthropometry, blood analytes and physical activity), to be published in summer 2003;

(iv)   Summary report, providing a summary of the key findings from the four volumes, to be published in autumn 2003.

2   The Technical Report is available online at http//www.food.gov.uk/science/(verified November 2002).

3   For further information about the archived data contact:
   The Data Archive
   University of Essex
   Wivenhoe Park
   Colchester
   Essex CO4 3SQ
   UK

   Tel: (UK) 01206 872001
   Fax: (UK) 01206 872003
   E-mail: archive@essex.ac.uk
   Website: www.data-archive.ac.uk

4   Responsibility for this survey and the National Diet and Nutrition Survey programme transferred from the Ministry of Agriculture, Fisheries and Food to the Food Standards Agency on its establishment in April 2000.

5   Gregory J, Foster K, Tyler H, Wiseman M. *The Dietary and Nutritional Survey of British Adults*. HMSO (London, 1990).

6   Finch S, Doyle W, Lowe C, Bates CJ, Prentice A, Smithers G, Clarke PC. *National Diet and Nutrition Survey: people aged 65 years and over. Volume 1: Report of the diet and nutrition survey*. TSO (London, 1998).

7   Gregory JR, Collins DL, Davies PSW, Hughes JM, Clarke PC. *National Diet and Nutrition Survey: children aged 1½ to 4½ years. Volume 1: Report of the diet and nutrition survey*. HMSO (London, 1995).

8   Gregory JR, Lowe S, Bates CJ, Prentice A, Jackson LV, Smithers G, Wenlock R, Farron M. *National Diet and Nutrition Survey: young people aged 4 to 18 years. Volume 1: Report of the diet and nutrition survey*. TSO (London, 2000).

9   Initially 30 addresses were selected within each postal sector. Results from Wave 1 indicated a higher level of age-related ineligibles than expected and a much lower response rate. In order to increase the actual number of diaries completed and to give interviewers enough work an extra 10 addresses were selected for Waves 2, 3 and 4.

10   The diet and physiology of pregnant or breastfeeding women is likely to be so different from those of other similarly aged women as to possibly distort the results. Further, as the number of pregnant or breastfeeding women identified within the overall sample of 2000 would not be adequate for analysis as a single group, it was decided that they should be regarded as ineligible for interview.

11   Selecting only one eligible adult per household reduces the burden of the survey on the household and therefore reduces possible detrimental effects on co-operation and data quality. It also reduces the clustering of the sample associated with similar dietary behaviour within the same household and improves the precision of the estimates.

12   As in some cases fieldwork extended beyond the end of the three-month fieldwork wave, or cases were re-allocated to another fieldwork wave, cases have been allocated to a wave for analysis purposes as follows. Any case started more than four weeks after the end of the official fieldwork wave has been allocated to the actual quarter in which it started. For example, all cases allocated to Wave 1 and started July to October 2000 appear as Wave 1 cases. Any case allocated to Wave 1 and started in November 2000 or later appears in a subsequent wave; for example a case allocated to Wave 1 which started in November 2000 is counted as Wave 2. All cases in Wave 4 (April to June 2001) had been started by the end of July 2001.

13   Initially 1,140 addresses were issued per wave. This was increased in Wave 2 to 1,520 addresses, 40 in each quota of work. In Wave 3, 27 addresses were withdrawn. These were unapproachable due to access restrictions in place because of the foot-and-mouth disease outbreak.

14   Martin J and Matheson J (1999) Responses to declining response rates on government surveys. *Survey Methodology Bulletin* 45, pp 33-7. July 1999.

15   Non-productive cases are those where the interviewer was unable to make contact with the selected household or respondent (non-contacts) and where the household or selected respondent refused to take part in the survey (refusals). Addresses that were returned to the office coded as refusals or non-contacts were considered for reissue. Where it was thought that a non-productive case might result in at least a dietary interview (for example, where the selected respondent had said they were too busy at the time of the original call but would be available at a later date) these addresses were issued to interviewers working in subsequent waves of fieldwork.

16 Skinner CJ and Holmes D (2001) *The 2000–01 National Diet and Nutrition Survey of Adults Aged 19–64 years: The Impact of Non-response.* University of Southampton. Reproduced as Appendix E of the Technical Report (*see* note 2).

Table 1.1

Response to the dietary interview and seven-day dietary record by wave of fieldwork*

Unweighted data
Numbers and percentages

| | **Wave of fieldwork** | | | | | | | | | **All** | |
| | Wave 1: July–September | | Wave 2: October–December | | Wave 3: January–March | | Wave 4: April–June | | | | |
	No.	%	No.	%	No.	%	No.	%	No.	%
Set sample = 100%	1098	100	1397	100	1450	100	1728	100	5673	100
Ineligible	382	35	514	37	515	36	558	32	1969	35
Eligible sample = 100%	716	100	883	100	935	100	1170	100	3704	100
Non-contacts	12	2	24	3	23	2	30	3	89	2
Refusals	271	38	369	42	364	39	360	31	1364	37
Co-operation with:										
dietary interview	433	60	490	56	548	59	780	67	2251	61
seven-day dietary record	325	45	385	44	429	46	585	50	1724	47

Note: * For productive cases, fieldwork wave is defined as the wave (quarter) in which the dietary interview took place; for unproductive cases, fieldwork wave is the wave in which the case was issued (or reissued).

2 Types and quantities of foods consumed

2.1 Introduction

This chapter presents data on the foods consumed by respondents in the survey. Most of the information is taken from the seven-day weighed intake dietary records, but some tables are based on information collected in the dietary interview; these include tables showing the consumption of artificial sweeteners, dietary supplements and milk, and whether the respondent reported being vegetarian or vegan.

2.2 Dietary interview data

2.2.1 Access to amenities

Nearly all the respondents taking part in the survey were living in households with a separate kitchen; only 1% of men and women were in accommodation with a shared kitchen. Most households had access to a range of amenities for the storage and preparation of food, such as a freezer, 96%, and microwave oven, 91%. Women aged 25 to 34 years were less likely than those aged 50 to 64 years to have access to a microwave oven (p<0.05). There were no other significant differences in access to amenities by age for men or women. For 88% of men and 85% of women the household had the use of a car or van. The proportions with access to a separate kitchen and to a freezer were close to those for a subsample of households from the 2000 General Household Survey (GHS)[1]. However, NDNS respondents were more likely than the 2000 GHS sample to have access to a microwave and a car or van (p<0.01).

(Table 2.1)

2.2.2 Current milk consumption

In the dietary interview[2], 45% of men and 56% of women said that they did not have milk as a drink (p<0.01). The proportions not drinking milk increased with age for both men and women. For men aged 19 to 24 years, 25% said they did not drink milk compared with 59% of those aged 50 to 64 years (p<0.01). For women, the proportion not drinking milk increased from 34% among the youngest age group to 51% among those aged 25 to 34 years, 57% among those aged 35 to 49 years and to 66% among those aged 50 to 64 years (19 to 24 years compared with 25 to 34: p<0.05; 19 to 24 years compared with 35 to 64: p<0.01).

Semi-skimmed cow's milk was reported as the usual milk for the highest proportion of men and women across all age groups. Men were more likely than women to report drinking semi-skimmed milk, 35% and 27% respectively, and whole milk, 18% and 12% (semi-skimmed milk: p<0.01; whole milk: p<0.05).

A much smaller proportion of respondents said that they did not have milk on cereal or in milk puddings than said they did not have milk as a drink: 18% of men and 13% of women said they never used milk on cereal or in puddings. Semi-skimmed milk was the usual milk used on cereals and in puddings for the highest proportion of men and women, 55% and 53% respectively. Whole milk was the usual milk for 22% of men and 19% of women, and skimmed for 7% and 16% respectively.

(Tables 2.2 and 2.3)

2.2.3 Artificial sweeteners

During the dietary interview, respondents were asked about their use of artificial sweeteners in tea, coffee and cooking. Overall, 5% of respondents reported using artificial sweeteners in tea, 6% in coffee, and 4% in cooking. Women were more likely than men to use artificial sweeteners in tea and in cooking (p<0.05). The highest reported use of artificial sweeteners was by women aged 50 to 64 years in coffee, 11% of whom used artificial sweeteners in this way.

The use of artificial sweeteners in tea by men increased with age, from none in the youngest age group to 4% among men aged 35 to 49, and to 6% among men aged 50 to 64 years (p<0.01). A similar pattern is evident for the use of artificial sweeteners in coffee for men, increasing from none in the youngest age group to 4% among those aged 25 to 34, and 5% among those aged 35 to 49 years, to 7% among the oldest group of men (19 to 24 compared with 25 to 34: p<0.05; 19 to 24 compared with 35 to 64: p<0.01). Women aged 19 to 24 years were less likely than the oldest group of women to have used artificial sweeteners in coffee, 3% and 11% respectively (p<0.05).

(Table 2.4)

2.2.4 Dietary supplements

Respondents were asked at the dietary interview if they were taking any extra vitamins, minerals, including fluoride, or other dietary supplements or herbal preparations, including prescribed or non-prescribed supplements. Those who reported taking supplements were asked to give a description of the product, including the brand name and strength, form, dose and frequency. Women were significantly more likely than men to report taking supplements; 40% and 29% respectively (p<0.01). Among women, 55% of those aged 50 to 64 years reported taking dietary supplements: this was higher than for all other groups of women (p<0.01). There were no other significant age-related trends.

The proportions taking supplements were higher among respondents from a non-manual than a manual home background for both men and women (p<0.01).

Of those taking supplements, cod liver oil and other fish-based supplements were taken by the highest proportion of respondents, 39%. Men were significantly more likely than women to be taking these types of supplements, 46% and

34% respectively (p<0.05). Multivitamins and multiminerals were taken by 35% of those taking supplements, 34% of men and 35% of women. Vitamin C only supplements were taken by 17% of respondents, as were non-nutrient supplements, such as ginseng, St Johns Wort, Echinacea and garlic. Overall, 14% of supplement-takers reported taking evening primrose oil-type supplements, but women were more likely to be taking these than men: 23% compared with 2% (p<0.01). Of supplement-takers, 12% reported taking multivitamins with no minerals, and the same proportion minerals only (excluding fluoride or iron only). Just under 10% of those who reported taking dietary supplements said they took vitamins with iron, and a similar proportion reported taking single vitamin supplements other than Vitamin C. Iron only supplements were taken by 2%, as were Vitamins A, C and D; fluoride supplements were taken by 1% of those taking supplements.

Prescribed folic acid was taken by 2%, and non-prescribed folic acid by 6%, of women taking supplements. Among women of childbearing age who were not pregnant and reported taking supplements, 10% of those aged 19 to 24, 7% of those aged 25 to 34, and 6% of those aged 35 to 49 years reported taking non-prescribed folic acid.

The youngest group of men and women were significantly less likely than those aged 50 to 64 years to be taking cod liver oil and other fish-based supplements (p<0.01). In addition, women aged 19 to 24 years were less likely than the oldest group to report taking evening primrose oil-type supplements, non-nutrient and 'other' types of supplements (evening primrose oil and 'other' supplements: p<0.05; non-nutrient supplements: p<0.01).

(Tables 2.5 and 2.6)

2.2.5 Dieting

All respondents were asked whether they were currently dieting to lose weight. Women were more likely to say they were dieting than men, with 24% of women and 10% of men reporting that, at the time of the interview, they were dieting to lose weight (p<0.01). Women aged 25 to 49 years were significantly more likely than men of the same age to report being on a diet (p<0.01). There were no significant age differences for men or women in the proportions who reported dieting to lose weight.

(Table 2.7)

2.2.6 Vegetarian/vegan

During the dietary interview, respondents were asked whether they were vegetarian or vegan. Overall, 5% of respondents reported being vegetarian or vegan. Women were more likely to report being vegetarian or vegan than men, 7% compared with 2% (p<0.01). The difference between men and women was most marked among those aged 25 to 34 years, where 11% of women but only 1% of men reported being vegetarian or vegan (p<0.01). The proportions showed almost no variation by age among men, but among women decreased significantly from about 11% among those aged 19 to 34, to about 4% among those aged 35 to 64 years (p<0.05). There were no differences in the proportion of respondents saying they were vegetarian or vegan by social class of the Household Reference Person (HRP).

Respondents who reported being vegetarian or vegan were asked what foods they avoided. All respondents said they avoided red meat, 92% avoided white meat and 48% did not eat fish. About one-third, 29%, said they avoided all animal products, and a fifth, 21%, said they avoided eating eggs.

Asked why they became vegetarian or vegan, 51% said it was for moral or ethical reasons, 29% for health reasons, and 25% because they did not like the taste of meat. Other less frequently mentioned reasons included religious beliefs, and cost or convenience. (Table not shown.)

Nearly two-thirds of respondents said they had never obtained any information about vegetarian and vegan diets. Of those that had obtained some information, the main sources were Vegetarian and Vegan Societies, or a doctor. Other less frequently mentioned sources of information included dietitians and nutritionists. (Table not shown.)

(Tables 2.8 and 2.9)

2.3 Foods consumed

2.3.1 Deriving food consumption data from the seven-day weighed intake dietary records

Every food item recorded in the dietary record, including those eaten away from home, was allocated an individual food code according to a coding frame based on 6,000 codes. This level of aggregation separates foods that are nutritionally different and, for some food types, separates at brand level. However, the data are more easily presented and interpreted when similar types of foods are grouped.

Each of the approximately 6,000 food codes used in the survey was allocated by the Food Standards Agency to one of 115 subsidiary food groups; these in turn can be aggregated into 57 food groups, and then into 11 food types. A complete list of food types, food groups and subsidiary food groups (with examples of the foods included in each subsidiary food group) is given in Appendix G of the Technical Report[3]. Consumption data for artificial sweeteners, dietary supplements and medicines are not shown in the tables since these items were recorded in tablets or teaspoons rather than as gram weights.

For each respondent completing a seven-day dietary record, the gram quantity of each food item consumed was calculated from the weight served and the weight, if any, left over. Food item data were then aggregated to subsidiary food group level and the total gram weight of all the items in the subsidiary food group consumed over the seven diary days was calculated. Diaries with fewer than seven days were excluded from the analysis.

The tables report consumption of most foods and drinks as served. Drinks that are made up with water such as instant coffee and dilutable squashes are recorded as the concentrate or powder/granules and water separately. In order to report consumption of these types of drinks as served, the tap water used as a diluent is coded in the same food group as the associated food. For example, water used to dilute low calorie fruit squash is coded to the low calorie concentrated soft drinks group. The consumption of tap water not used as a diluent is shown as a separate group in the tables. Tea and fresh coffee are recorded and reported as infusion. Where milk has been used to make up powdered beverages, the milk is coded to the appropriate milk group and the dry weight beverage to the beverages group. Thus the total fluid consumption of respondents can be estimated from the tables in this report.

The tables derived from the dietary records show the mean and median amounts of foods consumed in seven days for men and women separately, except for Table 2.14 which shows men and women combined. In Tables 2.11(a) and

2.11(b) these averages are based on *all* respondents who kept a dietary record, that is including both *consumers and non-consumers* of each food item. Other tables show mean and median amounts calculated for *consumers* of the item only and the percentage of respondents who consumed each item. Table 2.14 shows mean and median amounts consumed for all consumers and all respondents, for men and women combined.

2.3.2 Types of foods consumed by respondents and variation by sex

Tables 2.10(a) and (b) show the proportions of men and women consuming different foods during the seven-day dietary recording period. Table 2.10(c) summarises the differences between men and women, and the reader is referred to this table for the statistical significance levels of the differences commented on below.

The foods consumed by the largest proportions of respondents were: white bread, by 93% of men and 89% of women; savoury sauces, pickles, gravies & condiments, 94% and 91%; and 'other potatoes & potato dishes', for example boiled, mashed and jacket potatoes, 83% and 84%.

Within the cereal-based food group, white bread was consumed by the greatest proportion of respondents, 93% of men and 89% of women. This was followed by biscuits, which were consumed by 63% of men and 68% of women. More than half the men and women who completed a dietary record had eaten white bread, biscuits, buns, cakes & pastries, rice, pasta and 'other bread', for example brown bread, bagels and continental breads. Half the women had eaten whole grain & high fibre breakfast cereals. Wholemeal bread was consumed by 33% of men and 39% of women, and soft grain bread by 3% and 2% respectively. Men were more likely than women to have eaten white bread. There were no other significant differences in the proportion of men and women consuming cereal and cereal-based foods.

Nearly three-quarters of men and women, 74% and 73% respectively, consumed semi-skimmed milk, compared with just over a third, 36% and 35%, who consumed whole milk. Women were more likely than men to have had skimmed milk, 22% compared with 15%. Cheese other than cottage cheese was consumed by 78% of men

and 73% of women. Women were more likely than men to have eaten cottage cheese, fromage frais and yogurt. A higher proportion of men than women had eaten eggs during the recording period.

Butter was the most commonly consumed fat for spreading, consumed by 40% of men and 42% of women. This was followed by 'other', that is non-polyunsaturated reduced fat spreads, consumed by 37% of men and 33% of women. Men were more likely than women to have consumed non-polyunsaturated soft margarine, 32% compared with 23%. These proportions represent the use of fats as spreads, and do not include their use in cooking.

Chicken & turkey dishes were consumed by the largest proportion of respondents, 82% of men and 77% of women, followed by bacon & ham, eaten by 77% of men and 64% of women. Men were generally more likely to have eaten most types of meat and meat products than women (bacon & ham, beef, veal & dishes, pork & dishes, liver, liver products & dishes, burgers & kebabs, sausages, meat pies & pastries and 'other meat & meat products', for example game, haggis and corned beef). Indeed, the only meat products that men were no more likely than women to have eaten were coated chicken & turkey, chicken & turkey dishes and lamb & dishes.

Bananas were the most commonly consumed fruit, eaten by 49% of men and 56% of women, followed by apples & pears, which were eaten by 49% of men and 54% of women. During the seven-day recording period, only 25% of men and 30% of women recorded eating any citrus fruits. Women were more likely than men to have eaten 'other fruit', for example plums, grapes and soft fruits, 51% and 37% respectively.

The group of vegetables consumed by the greatest proportion of respondents was 'other vegetables', which includes, for example, mushrooms, cauliflower, onions and peppers, eaten by 81% of men and 80% of women, and 'other raw' & salad vegetables, excluding raw tomatoes and raw carrots, eaten by 76% and 81% respectively. Raw tomatoes were eaten by 67% of men and 70% of women, leafy green vegetables by 49% and 56%, cooked carrots by 57% and 56%, and peas by 59% of men and 52% of women. Men were more likely than women to have eaten baked beans, 48% and 41% respectively. There were no other significant differences between men and women in the proportions consuming specific types of vegetables.

'Other potatoes & potato dishes', for example boiled, mashed and jacket potatoes, were consumed by 83% of men and 84% of women. The next most commonly consumed potato-based item was potato chips, eaten by a higher proportion of men than women, 75% compared with 67%. Savoury snacks were eaten by 55% of men and 57% of women.

Over half of all respondents, 54% of men and 57% of women, had eaten chocolate confectionery during the seven-day dietary recording period, and about a fifth, 20% of men and 25% of women, had eaten sugar confectionery. Men were more likely than women to have consumed table sugar, 60% compared with 48%. The difference in the use of table sugar may be associated with the differences between the sexes in their reported use of sugar in tea and in coffee (see Table 2.4, page 00).

Among soft drinks, men and women were most likely to have drunk carbonated soft drinks not low calorie, 52% and 42%, and fruit juice, 43% of men and 47% of women. While men were more likely than women to have drunk carbonated soft drinks not low calorie, women were more likely than men to have drunk low calorie carbonated soft drinks.

Beer & lager were the most commonly consumed alcoholic drinks among men, drunk by 66%, but less commonly by women, 24%. For women, wine was the most commonly consumed alcoholic drink, with 45% drinking this compared with 36% of men. In addition to these differences, men were more likely than women to have drunk cider & perry, while women were more likely to have drunk liqueurs and alco-pops.

Both tea and coffee were drunk by nearly three-quarters of respondents, tea by 77% of both men and women, and coffee by 72% of men and 70% of women. A significantly higher proportion of women than men recorded drinking herbal tea, tap water and 'other beverages', for example, drinking chocolate and malted drinks.

(Tables 2.10(a), (b) and (c))

2.3.3 Variation in the foods eaten by age group

The data clearly show that there were differences in the foods consumed by respondents in different age groups (see Tables 2.10(a) and (b)

and, for a summary of the differences, with significance values, Table 2.10(c)).

The greatest age differences in foods consumed for men and women is between those aged 19 to 24 years and those aged 50 to 64 years. The discussion will focus on the foods consumed by these two age groups.

Men and women aged 19 to 24 years were more likely than those aged 50 to 64 to have consumed coated chicken & turkey, burgers & kebabs, savoury snacks, carbonated soft drinks not low calorie and alco-pops. For example, nearly two-thirds of men, and one-third of women, aged 19 to 24 years had eaten burgers & kebabs during the recording period, compared with one in ten of the oldest group of men and women. The proportion drinking alco-pops decreased from 21% of women and 16% of men aged 19 to 24 years, to 2% of women and none of the men aged 50 to 64 years. The proportion drinking carbonated soft drinks not low calorie, decreased from 92% and 64% of men and women aged 19 to 24 to 33% and 32% of those aged 50 to 64.

In addition, the youngest group of men was more likely than men aged 50 to 64 to have consumed pasta, pizza and potato chips; and the youngest group of women was more likely than the oldest group to have drunk concentrated soft drinks, both low calorie and not low calorie, and beer & lager.

A much greater number of foods were less likely to have been eaten by the youngest age group than the oldest age group. For nearly half of the fruit and vegetable types (peas, leafy green vegetables, tomatoes not raw, apples & pears, citrus fruits, bananas, canned fruit in juice and 'other fruit' – for example plums, grapes and soft fruits) a significantly lower proportion of men and women aged 19 to 24 years had consumed the item compared with the oldest age group. For example, 30% of men and 43% of women aged 19 to 24 years had consumed leafy green vegetables compared with 64% of men and 70% of women aged 50 to 64 years. In the youngest age group, 25% of men and 28% of women had consumed bananas compared with 59% of men and 69% of women in the oldest age group. Additionally, among men, those in the youngest age group were less likely than those in the oldest age group to have eaten raw carrots, green beans, and 'other potato & potato dishes', for example boiled, mashed and jacket potatoes.

Women aged 19 to 24 years were less likely than those aged 50 to 64 years to have eaten raw tomatoes, cooked carrots and canned fruit in syrup.

Other foods that were less likely to have been consumed by the youngest group of men and women compared with the oldest group were wholemeal bread, whole grain & high fibre breakfast cereals, fruit pies, eggs, oily fish, preserves, low alcohol & alcohol free beer & lager, and coffee. For example, 18% of men and 38% of women aged 19 to 24 had consumed oily fish compared with 54% of men and 58% of women aged 50 to 64 years. The youngest group of men was also less likely than those aged 50 to 64 years to have consumed 'other cereal-based puddings' (for example trifle and cheesecakes), whole and skimmed milk, cottage cheese, pork & pork dishes, liver, liver products & liver dishes and wine. Women aged 19 to 24 years were less likely than those aged 50 to 64 years to have eaten buns, cakes & pastries, cream, egg dishes, coated and/or fried white fish, 'other white fish & fish dishes' and soup, and to have drunk fortified wine and herbal tea.

(Tables 2.10(a), (b) and (c))

2.3.4 Quantities of foods consumed

Tables 2.11(a) and (b) show the average (mean) quantities of foods consumed by all respondents in the survey. In these tables the means are calculated including non-consumers: those who did not record consuming any of the food during the seven-day dietary recording period. The data are shown separately for men and women within the four age bands. Table 2.11(c) summarises the differences between men and women in average amounts eaten, and shows significance values.

For many food items, men ate significantly larger mean amounts than women. In all age groups, men consumed larger mean amounts of bacon & ham and beer & lager than women in the same age group. For example, among those aged 19 to 24 years, men consumed an average of 125g of bacon & ham during the seven-day recording period compared with 62g by women. Indeed, within each age group, men consumed almost twice as much bacon & ham as women. Among those aged 50 to 64 years, men consumed 2357g of beer & lager, almost 16 times as much as consumed by women (145g). From the age of 25 years, men consumed a larger mean amount of white bread, eggs, chicken & turkey dishes,

meat pies & pastries, sausages, potato chips and table sugar than women from the same age group. There were relatively few foods that were consumed in greater quantities by women than by men. Women, apart from those aged 25 to 34 years, ate significantly larger mean amounts of 'other fruit', for example plums, grapes and soft fruits, than the same aged men.

(Tables 2.11(a), (b) and (c))

Tables 2.10(a) and (b) give mean and median consumption figures based only on those consuming the food item: 'consumers'. For a number of food items in this NDNS, the actual number of respondents consuming the item is too small to allow reliable interpretation of mean values and results of significance tests of differences in mean amounts consumed. Differences in the amounts consumed by those aged 19 to 24 years compared with those aged 50 to 64 years were, therefore, assessed for statistical significance for only those food items consumed by at least 30 respondents in both age groups.

Compared with the oldest group of men and women, consumers aged 19 to 24 years ate significantly larger mean amounts of potato chips, and consumed more than double the amount of savoury snacks and carbonated soft drinks not low calorie ($p < 0.01$). For example, the youngest group of men and women respectively consumed 528g and 434g of potato chips during the dietary recording period compared with 341g and 247g by those aged 50 to 64 years. In addition, the youngest men consumed at least double the mean amount of pizza and baked beans than those aged 50 to 64 years; and the youngest group of women consumed more pasta than the oldest group of women ($p < 0.01$).

Conversely, men and women aged 50 to 64 years consumed significantly larger mean amounts of buns, cakes & pastries, semi-skimmed milk, 'other raw' & salad vegetables (excluding raw tomatoes and raw carrots), leafy green vegetables, 'other vegetables' (for example, mushrooms, cauliflower, onions and peppers), apples & pears and tea than those aged 19 to 24 years (buns, cakes & pastries and 'other raw' & salad vegetables: $p < 0.05$; all others: $p < 0.01$). For example, the oldest group of men and women consumed 498g and 482g respectively of apples & pears during the dietary recording period compared with 251g and 283g by those aged 19 to 24 years. The amount of tea consumed by the oldest group of men and women was more than double that consumed by the youngest group. In addition, the oldest group of men consumed significantly larger mean amounts of raw tomatoes, peas, cooked carrots, 'other potatoes & potato dishes' (for example boiled, mashed and jacket potatoes) and table sugar than those aged 19 to 24 years (peas: $p<0.05$; all others: $p<0.01$). Compared to the youngest group of women, the oldest group consumed significantly larger mean amounts of whole grain & high fibre breakfast cereals and butter (whole grain & high fibre breakfast cereals: $p<0.05$; butter: $p<0.01$).

Generally, the food items eaten in significantly larger amounts by the youngest group of men and women were also more likely to be eaten by this age group than by those aged 50 to 64 years. The same pattern was true for those food items eaten in significantly larger amounts by the oldest group of men and women.

(Tables 2.10(a) and (b))

2.3.5 Variation in the foods eaten by region

Tables 2.12(a) and (b) show the proportions of men and women in each region who consumed different types of food in the seven-day dietary recording period[4]. There were differences, for both men and women, in the proportions consuming different foods according to the region in which they lived: the greatest number of significant differences was between respondents living in London and the South East and those living in other regions. There were, however, no consistent differences in eating patterns between regions. For example, respondents in no one region were more likely to have consumed cereal and cereal-based products and less likely to have consumed fruit and vegetables than those in other regions. The main differences between regions are summarised in Table 2.12(c), and the reader is referred to this table for regional comparisons of differences and significance values. The commentary reports on the foods that show the most marked differences ($p<0.01$) in consumption by men and women in the different regions. The reader should note that the sample size in Scotland is particularly low and, therfore, standard errors may be large (for further details on standard errors, *see* Appendix B, page 69–73).

Women living in Scotland were more likely than all other women to have consumed soup. For example, 70% of women in Scotland had consumed soup compared with 30% of women in Central and South West regions of England and in Wales. Men living in Scotland were more likely than those in the Northern region, and in Central and South West regions of England and in Wales to have drunk tap water during the dietary recording period.

Men living in the Northern region were more likely than those in London and the South East to have eaten meat pies & pastries. Women in the Northern region were more likely, along with those in Central and South West regions of England and in Wales, and London and the South East, to have consumed 'other cereals', for example bran, oats and Yorkshire puddings, compared with women in Scotland.

A significantly higher proportion of men living in Central and South West regions of England and in Wales ate potato chips than those in London and the South East, and drank concentrated soft drinks not low calorie compared with men in Scotland. Men in this region, and those in London and the South East, were also more likely than those in Scotland to have consumed 'other milk', for example soya milk, evaporated and condensed milk. Women living in Central and South West regions of England and in Wales were more likely than those in Scotland to have eaten peas.

Men living in London and the South East were more likely to have consumed butter than those in the Northern region, and bottled water and vegetable dishes compared with men in any other region. They were also more likely to have consumed nuts & seeds than men in Scotland, and 'other bread', for example brown bread, bagels and continental breads, compared with men in the Northern region, and in Central and South West regions of England and in Wales. Women living in London and the South East were more likely to have consumed vegetable dishes, green beans and nuts & seeds, and to have drunk herbal tea, compared with those in the Northern region.

(Tables 2.12(a), (b) and (c))

2.3.6 Variation in the foods eaten by household receipt of benefits

Tables 2.13(a) and (b) show the proportions of respondents consuming different types of food, and the mean and median amounts consumed according to whether the household was in receipt of certain state benefits[5]. The principal differences in the foods consumed by respondents, according to whether the household was in receipt of benefits or not, are summarised in Table 2.13(c), and the reader is referred to this table for the statistical significance of the differences commented on below.

Overall, Table 2.13(c) shows clearly that there is a comparatively wide range of foods that were less likely to have been eaten by respondents from benefit households. In contrast there are relatively few foods that respondents from benefit households were more likely to eat compared with those living in non-benefit households. There are also more differences by household benefit status for women than men.

Table sugar was the only food item to have been consumed by a higher proportion of both men and women in benefit households compared with those in non-benefit households. This was consumed by 74% of men and 58% of women in benefit households, and by 58% of men and 46% of women in non-benefit households. Additionally, women living in benefit households were more likely than women in non-benefit households to have consumed whole milk, 49% and 32%, burgers & kebabs, 27% and 16%, and meat pies & pastries, 44% and 30%.

The number of foods that were less likely to have been eaten by those in benefit households than those in non-benefit households was much greater. For both men and women, soft grain bread, 'other bread' (for example brown bread, bagels and continental breads), whole grain & high fibre breakfast cereals, cream, cottage cheese, yogurt, shellfish, and oily fish were less likely to have been consumed by those in benefit households than those in non-benefit households. Additionally, a lower proportion of women in households in receipt of benefits had consumed pasta, wholemeal bread, biscuits, buns, cakes & pastries, 'other cereal-based puddings' (for example trifle and cheesecakes), skimmed milk, cheese other than cottage cheese, ice cream, butter and other oils & cooking fats not polyunsaturated. The only type of meat and meat product to show any difference by household benefit status was chicken & turkey dishes, with men in benefit households less likely to have consumed this than those in non-benefit households.

Respondents from households receiving benefits were less likely to have eaten many types of fruit and vegetables than respondents from non-benefit households. Both men and women in benefit households were less likely than those in non-benefit households to have eaten 'other raw' & salad vegetables (that is excluding raw tomatoes and raw carrots), leafy green vegetables, vegetable dishes, apples & pears, bananas and 'other fruit', for example plums, grapes and soft fruits. Additionally a lower proportion of men from households in receipt of benefits recorded eating nuts & seeds and drinking fruit juice, than did men from non-benefit households. Raw carrots, raw tomatoes, green beans, cooked carrots, 'other vegetables' (for example, mushrooms, cauliflower, onions and peppers) and citrus fruits were less likely to have been eaten by women in benefit households than those in households not in receipt of benefits. Indeed, among women the only fruit and vegetables that were no less likely to have been consumed by benefit households were peas, baked beans, tomatoes not raw, and fruit in fruit juice or syrup.

The proportion of men and women who had drunk wine was significantly lower for those in households in receipt of benefits compared with those in non-benefit households, as was the proportion of men and women who had drunk bottled water and tap water. Compared with those in non-benefit households, men in benefit households were also less likely to have drunk fortified wine, beer & lager and herbal teas; women from benefit households were less likely to have had low calorie carbonated soft drinks and 'other beverages', for example drinking chocolate and malted drinks.

(Tables 2.13(a), (b) and (c))

2.4 Fruit and vegetables consumed

2.4.1 Introduction

Earlier in the chapter we looked at consumption of fruit and vegetables at the subsidiary food group level (see sections 2.3.1 to 2.3.6). This gave information on the proportion of respondents who consumed different types of fruit and vegetables, and the mean and median amounts consumed over the seven-day dietary recording period. This section looks at the number of portions, and the mean and median amounts of all fruit and all vegetables consumed daily.

2.4.2 Background

Government initiative.

A key feature of the Government's framework for reducing early deaths from coronary heart disease and cancer, and reducing health inequalities among the general population is to improve access to and increase the consumption of fruit and vegetables. The World Health Organization (WHO) and the UK's Committee on Medical Aspects of Food and Nutrition (COMA) policy recommend eating at least five portions (400g) of fruit and vegetables a day. This recommendation forms the basis of the five-a-day programme, part of the action intended to achieve these targets[6].

Information collected by the NDNS allows the analysis of consumption of fruit and vegetables among British adults aged 19 to 64, and provides a baseline for evaluating the impact of the five-a-day programme among this age group.

2.4.3 Deriving fruit and vegetable consumption data from the seven-day weighed intake dietary records

Fruit and vegetable consumption in the NDNS sample is examined using the definition of fruit and vegetables used within the five-a-day programme. Thus, most fruit and vegetables count, but starchy, staple vegetables, such as potatoes, yams and cassavas, do not. Fruit and vegetable juices count, as do pulses and beans, but not rice. Fresh, cooked, frozen, chilled, canned and dried forms of fruit and vegetables all count, as do fruit and vegetables in selected composite dishes, such as stews and fruit pies.

Given the detailed information collected about fruit and vegetable consumption in the NDNS, it is possible to construct a number of variables to describe fruit and vegetable consumption. The main analytic variable, which is shown in the tables and on which the commentary mainly focuses, is:

> Daily consumption of fruit and vegetables, including those in selected composite dishes[7]: including all fruit juice consumed as one portion only and, similarly all baked beans and other pulses consumed as one portion only[8].

Additional variables have been calculated. These consider fruit and vegetables separately, with and without composite dishes. Variables have been calculated for fruit to: (i) exclude fruit juice; (ii) count all fruit juice consumed as one portion only; and (iii) count all portions of fruit juice.

Variables for vegetables have been calculated to: (i) exclude baked beans and other pulses; (ii) count all baked beans and other pulses consumed as one portion only; and (iii) count all portions of baked beans and other pulses. Appendix A (*see* page 51–68) gives more detail on the derivation of these variables. Tables showing the proportions consuming fruit and vegetables, and the quantities consumed for all variables by sex and age, region, and household receipt of benefits are also given in Appendix A (Tables A2(a) to A8). It is possible to see from these tables the proportions of respondents who ate fruit, the proportions who ate vegetables, and the differences that the inclusion of composite dishes, and all portions of fruit juice and baked beans and other pulses, make to the amounts of fruit and vegetables consumed daily.

The recommendation is that five portions or 400g of fruit and vegetables are consumed daily. This equates to approximately 80g per portion[9], and is the definition of a 'portion' used in these analyses. For composite fruit dishes, only fruit pies have been included, not other fruit dishes such as fruit crumbles and yogurts: for fruit pies, the fruit contribution has been estimated as 45% of the total weight consumed. For composite vegetable dishes, the vegetable contribution has been estimated as 40% of the total weight consumed.

2.4.4 Portions of fruit and vegetables consumed

Tables 2.15(a) to 2.17(c) show distributions and the average (mean) number of portions of fruit and vegetables, including composite dishes, consumed in a day for all respondents including non-consumers. Tables 2.15(a), 2.16(a) and 2.17(a) show portions for fruit and vegetables combined, including all fruit juice consumed as one portion only and all baked beans and other pulses consumed as one portion only. Tables 2.15(b), 2.16(b) and 2.17(b) show portions of fruit, including all fruit juice consumed as one portion only, and Tables 2.15(c), 2.16(c) and 2.17(c) show portions of vegetables, including all baked beans and other pulses consumed as one portion only.

2.4.5 Portions of fruit and vegetables consumed by sex and age of respondent

Table 2.15(a) shows the average number of portions of fruit and vegetables consumed daily by sex and age, Table 2.15(b) shows the average number of portions of fruit only, and Table 2.15(c) vegetables only.

On average, men and women consumed fewer than three portions of fruit and vegetables a day: 2.7 for men and 2.9 for women (medians 2.2 and 2.4). The portions consumed comprise an average of around one and a half portions of fruit, 1.3 for men and 1.5 for women (medians 0.9 and 1.0) and one and a half portions of vegetables a day, 1.4 and 1.4 respectively (medians 1.2 and 1.2). There were no significant differences in the mean number of portions of fruit, vegetables, or fruit and vegetables combined consumed by sex.

For both men and women, those aged 19 to 24 years consumed a lower mean number of portions of fruit and vegetables combined than those aged 50 to 64 years (p<0.01). For example, the youngest men consumed an average of 1.3 portions of fruit and vegetables a day during the recording period, compared with 3.6 portions by the oldest group of men (medians 1.3 and 3.4). The youngest group of women consumed an average of 1.8 portions of fruit and vegetables, while those aged 50 to 64 consumed an average of 3.8 portions (medians 1.6 and 3.3). This age difference in the mean number of portions consumed was also true for fruit and vegetables when considered separately (p<0.01).

Generally median values are much lower than mean values, indicating that mean values are affected by the relatively small number of respondents who ate lots of fruit and vegetables. For example, the mean and median number of portions of fruit and vegetables consumed by men were 2.7 and 2.2 respectively.

Overall, 13% of men and 15% of women consumed five or more portions of fruit and vegetables a day. Only 1% of men and none of the women who kept a seven-day dietary record consumed five or more portions of vegetables, and 3% of both men and women consumed five or more portions of fruit a day.

The proportion of men and women eating five or more portions of fruit and vegetables a day increased with age. For example, none of the men and 4% of women aged 19 to 24 years had consumed five or more portions of fruit and vegetables, compared with 24% of men and 22% of women aged 50 to 64 years (p<0.01).

When fruit and vegetables are considered separately, it is evident that the age differences in the proportions consuming five or more portions

of fruit and vegetables derive mainly from differences in the consumption of fruit (see Tables 2.15(b) and 2.15(c)). For example, men aged 19 to 34 years were less likely than those aged 50 to 64 years to have consumed five or more portions of fruit (25 to 34: p<0.05; 19 to 24: p<0.01). Women aged 19 to 24 years were less likely than those aged 35 to 64 to have had at least five portions of fruit a day (35 to 49: p<0.05; 50 to 64: p<0.01). There were no age differences in the proportions who had consumed five or more portions of vegetables.

Overall, only 1% of men and women recorded eating no fruit or vegetables during the seven-day dietary recording period and only 2% no vegetables. There were no significant age differences in the proportions that had eaten no fruit or vegetables. This was also true for vegetables alone. However, there were differences in the proportions that had consumed no fruit. Over one fifth, 21%, of men had eaten no fruit during the seven-day dietary recording period, compared with 15% of women (p<0.05). The proportion of men who had eaten no fruit during the dietary recording period declined with age, from 45% of those aged 19 to 24 years to 11% of those aged 50 to 64 years (p<0.01). A similar pattern is evident for women, with 27% of the youngest group and 5% of the oldest group having eaten no fruit (p<0.01).

(Tables 2.15(a), (b) and (c))

2.4.6 Portions of fruit and vegetables consumed by region

Tables 2.16(a) to 2.16(c) show the average number of portions of fruit and vegetables consumed by region. There were no significant regional differences for men or women in the mean number of portions of fruit and vegetables consumed. The mean number of portions consumed ranged from 2.6 for men and 2.7 for women in the Northern region, to 3.0 and 3.2 respectively for men and women living in London and the South East. There were also no significant differences by region in the mean number of portions of fruit consumed. However, women living in London and the South East consumed a higher mean number of portions of vegetables than women in Scotland and the Northern region (Northern: p<0.05; Scotland: p<0.01).

There were no significant regional differences in the proportion of men and women who consumed five or more portions of fruit and vegetables a day, or in the proportion who had eaten no fruit and vegetables. This was also true when consumption of fruit and vegetables were considered separately.

(Tables 2.16(a), (b) and (c))

2.4.7 Portions of fruit and vegetables consumed by household receipt of benefits

Table 2.17(a) shows that men and women living in households in receipt of state benefits consumed a significantly lower mean number of portions of fruit and vegetables than those in non-benefit households. For example, men in benefit households consumed an average of 2.1 portions of fruit and vegetables a day, compared with 2.8 by men in non-benefit households (p<0.05). Women in benefit households consumed an average of 1.9 portions of fruit and vegetables a day, compared with 3.1 portions for women in non-benefit households (p<0.01).

Women in benefit households were less likely than those in non-benefit households to have consumed five or more portions of fruit and vegetables a day: 4% and 17% respectively (p<0.01). There was no significant difference for men by household benefit status.

When considering fruit and vegetables separately, there were no significant differences by benefit status in the proportion of men and women who consumed five or more portions of either fruit or vegetables. However, women in benefit households did consume a lower mean number of portions of vegetables than those in non-benefit households (p<0.01).

About a third, 35% of men and 30% of women, in benefit households had eaten no fruit during the seven-day dietary recording period, compared with 19% and 12% of men and women in non-benefit households (men: p<0.05; women: p<0.01). A much smaller proportion had eaten no vegetables: 4% of men and 6% of women in benefit households, and 2% of men and 1% of women in non-benefit households (men: ns; women: p<0.05).

(Tables 2.17(a), (b) and (c))

References and endnotes

[1] The General Household Survey (GHS) is a multi-purpose continuous survey carried out by the Social Survey Division of the Office for National Statistics (ONS) which collects information on a range of topics from people living in private households in Great Britain. The 2000 GHS was carried out between April 2000 and March 2001: the set sample size was 13,250, and the response rate was 67%. Comparison data is from households containing at least one person aged 19 to 64 years: 6,411 unweighted, and 19,572,762 weighted and grossed.

[2] The interview questionnaire is reproduced in Appendix A of the Technical Report, which can be found at http//www.food.gov.uk/science (verified November 2002).

[3] The subsidiary food groups include infant formula, commercial infant drinks and commercial infant foods; none of the respondents in the survey consumed any of the food items in these subgroups in the seven-day recording period and therefore these subsidiary food groups are omitted from the tables. Examples of the foods included in each subsidiary food is given in Appendix G of the Technical Report, available online at http//www.food.gov.uk/science/ (verified November 2002).

[4] The areas included in each of the four analysis 'regions' are given in the response chapter, Chapter 2 of the Technical Report, online at http//www.food.gov.uk/science (verified November 2002). Definitions of 'regions' are given in the glossary (see Appendix D).

[5] Households receiving benefits are those where someone in the respondent's household was currently receiving Working Families Tax Credit or had, in the previous 14 days, drawn Income Support or (Income-related) Job Seeker's Allowance. Definitions of 'household' and 'benefits (receiving)' are given in the glossary (see Appendix D).

[6] The five-a-day programme is being developed by the Department of Health, in conjunction with the Food Standards Agency, the Department of the Environment, Food and Rural Affairs (DEFRA), the Department for Education and Skills (DfES) and the Health Development Agency. Consumer, health, education and parent organisations are also involved along with the food industry. More information can be obtained online at http://www.doh.gov.uk/fiveaday/(verified November 2002).

[7] Composite dishes included in the analysis of fruit and vegetable consumption were: for fruit, fruit pies; and for vegetables, vegetable dishes (including vegetable lasagne, cauliflower cheese and vegetable samosas). See also Appendix A.

[8] Part of the recommendations is that a variety of fruit and vegetables should be eaten. It would be relatively easy to consume 3 to 4 glasses of fruit juice a day, providing five portions, but this would not encourage the variety in intake that is recommended.

[9] In calculating compliance with Government recommendations to eat at least five portions of a variety of fruit and vegetables a day, a glass (150ml) of fruit or vegetable juice is considered one portion. Fruit or vegetable juice can only contribute one portion towards five-a-day, even if more than one glass of 100% is consumed. The portion size of fruit juice used for these analyses was 80g. However, the analyses in this chapter are based on the definition of fruit and vegetables in which all fruit juice consumed in a day (one portion of or over) is counted as one portion only, the use of 80g or 150ml to define a portion will have little impact on the results in terms of measuring compliance with Government recommendations.

Table 2.1

Household access to amenities and domestic appliances

Responding sample Percentages

Amenities and domestic appliances	Men aged (years):				All men	Women aged (years):				All women	All NDNS	GHS2000*
	19–24	25–34	35–49	50–64		19–24	25–34	35–49	50–64			
With a separate kitchen	100	99	99	100	99	99	99	99	100	99	99	100**
Owns or has use of:												
refrigerator	98	96	97	97	97	98	97	95	97	96	96	..
deep freezer or fridge freezer	95	96	96	95	96	96	96	97	97	97	96	95
microwave oven	89	89	92	90	90	89	87	92	94	91	91	86
car or van	79	90	90	89	88	78	82	89	85	85	86	80
Base	*142*	*287*	*330*	*330*	*1088*	*136*	*275*	*415*	*337*	*1163*	*2251*	*6411*

Note: * 2000 General Household Survey: weighted data from a subsample of households containing at least one adult aged 19 to 64 years.
** General Household Survey data on separate kitchens refers to those households with a separate kitchen not in a bedsit.
.. Does not apply; not asked in the General Household Survey.

Table 2.2

Type of milk respondent usually had as a drink by sex and age of respondent

Responding sample Percentages

Type of milk respondent usually had as a drink	Men aged (years):				All men	Women aged (years):				All women	All
	19–24	25–34	35–49	50–64		19–24	25–34	35–49	50–64		
Did not have milk as a drink	25	35	49	59	45	34	51	57	66	56	51
Whole cow's milk	29	24	13	11	18	19	14	12	9	12	15
Semi-skimmed cow's milk	45	40	35	26	35	42	29	26	20	27	31
Skimmed cow's milk	2	4	4	5	4	5	6	7	6	6	5
Powdered milk	-	-	-	-	-	-	-	0	0	0	0
Soya alternative (soya milk)	-	-	-	-	-	-	1	-	-	0	0
Goat's milk	-	0	-	-	0	-	-	0	0	0	0
Other type of milk	2	1	1	0	1	-	1	0	-	0	1
*Base**	*142*	*287*	*330*	*330*	*1088*	*136*	*275*	*415*	*337*	*1163*	*2251*

Note: * Percentages add to more than 100 as some respondents usually drank more than one type of milk.

Table 2.3

Type of milk respondent usually used on breakfast cereal and in puddings by sex and age of respondent

Responding sample Percentages

Type of milk respondent usually had on cereal and in puddings	Men aged (years):				All men	Women aged (years):				All women	All
	19–24	25–34	35–49	50–64		19–24	25–34	35–49	50–64		
Did not have any milk	23	16	17	16	18	16	14	13	12	13	15
Whole cow's milk	22	28	18	22	22	22	20	20	16	19	21
Semi-skimmed cow's milk	54	51	60	53	55	57	51	53	54	53	54
Skimmed cow's milk	2	6	7	10	7	6	16	17	19	16	12
Powdered milk	-	-	0	1	0	-	0	-	0	0	0
Soya alternative (soya milk)	-	1	-	0	0	-	1	1	2	1	1
Other type of milk	-	-	0	-	0	-	1	1	0	1	0
*Base**	*142*	*287*	*330*	*330*	*1088*	*136*	*275*	*415*	*337*	*1163*	*2251*

Note: * Percentages add to more than 100 as some respondents for example, usually had more than one type of milk on cereal.

Table 2.4

Use of sugar and artificial sweeteners by sex and age of respondent

Responding sample   Percentages

Use of sugar and artificial sweeteners	Men aged (years):				All men	Women aged (years):				All women	All
	19–24	25–34	35–49	50–64		19–24	25–34	35–49	50–64		
Tea drinking											
Drinks tea:											
with sugar	61	42	41	34	42	37	27	22	17	24	32
with artificial sweetener	-	3	4	6	4	4	5	8	9	7	5
unsweetened	21	35	43	48	39	37	48	54	60	52	46
Does not drink tea	18	20	13	12	15	22	20	16	14	17	16
Coffee drinking											
Drinks coffee:											
with sugar	53	49	44	41	46	31	28	24	27	27	36
with artificial sweetener	-	4	5	7	5	3	5	9	11	8	6
unsweetened	11	35	36	37	33	22	36	49	48	42	38
Does not drink coffee	36	12	16	15	17	44	31	18	14	23	20
In cooking											
Uses artificial sweeteners	1	3	3	4	3	3	6	6	7	6	4
Base	*142*	*287*	*330*	*330*	*1088*	*136*	*275*	*415*	*337*	*1163*	*2251*

Table 2.5

Whether respondent reported currently taking dietary supplements (including fluoride) by sex and age of respondent and social class of household reference person

Responding sample   Percentages

	Percentage taking supplements*	*Base*
Sex and age of respondent		
Men aged (years):		
19–24	22	*142*
25–34	28	*287*
35–49	29	*330*
50–64	34	*330*
All men	29	*1088*
Women aged (years):		
19–24	31	*136*
25–34	34	*275*
35–49	36	*415*
50–64	55	*337*
All women	40	*1163*
Sex of respondent and social class of household reference person		
Men:		
Non-manual	35	*603*
Manual	22	*460*
All men**	29	*1088*
Women:		
Non-manual	49	*631*
Manual	30	*486*
All women**	40	*1163*
All	35	*2251*

Note: * Includes women taking prescribed folic acid.
       **Includes those for whom a social class could not be assigned.

Table 2.6

Dietary supplements reported in the dietary interview as being taken by sex and age of respondent

Those reporting in the dietary interview taking supplements

Percentages*

Dietary supplement	Men aged (years):				All men	Women aged (years):				All women	All
	19–24	25–34	35–49	50–64		19–24	25–34	35–49	50–64		
Fluoride only	-	2	-	1	1	-	-	1	-	0	1
Cod liver oil and other fish-based supplements	[2]	43	45	59	46	13	10	32	53	34	39
Evening primrose oil type supplements	-	1	3	2	2	7	18	26	27	23	14
Vitamin C only	[1]	16	23	20	18	20	19	18	14	17	17
Other single vitamins, not vitamin C	-	3	9	7	6	10	10	9	13	11	9
Vitamins A, C and D only	-	2	-	1	1	10	5	4	1	3	2
Vitamins with iron	[6]	4	9	8	8	20	11	6	5	8	8
Iron only	-	-	3	2	2	3	4	3	1	2	2
Prescribed folic acid**	..	..	..	..	..	1	1	2	2	2	..
Non-prescribed folic acid only	-	-	-	1	0	10	7	6	4	6	3
Multivitamins and multiminerals	[11]	44	31	28	34	25	37	40	32	35	35
Multivitamins, no minerals	[1]	15	17	8	12	17	7	10	12	11	12
Minerals only, not fluoride or iron only	[1]	6	12	8	9	8	7	10	24	15	12
Non-nutrient supplements***	[1]	8	12	24	15	5	15	19	25	19	17
Other****	[10]	10	7	17	14	10	21	17	30	22	19
Base	27	79	93	108	306	40	88	145	171	444	750

Note: * Percentages add up to more than 100 as some respondents were taking more than one type of supplement.
 ** Square brackets enclosing numbers denote the actual numbers of cases, when the base is fewer than 30.
 *** This was asked in a separate question of women only.
 **** This includes: ginseng, ginkgo, garlic, St Johns Wort, Aloe, Saw Palmetto, Red Clover, Hawthorn, Echinacea, Goldenseal, and Echinacea and Goldenseal.
 ***** This includes, for example, glucosamine sulphate, royal jelly and milk thistle.

Table 2.7

Percentage of respondents who reported dieting to lose weight by sex and age of respondent

Responding sample

Percentages

	Percentage reporting dieting to lose weight	Base
Sex and age of respondent		
Men aged (years):		
19–24	9	142
25–34	6	287
35–49	12	330
50–64	13	330
All men	10	1088
Women aged (years):		
19–24	21	136
25–34	28	275
35–49	25	415
50–64	20	337
All women	24	1163
All	17	2251

Table 2.8

Percentage of respondents who reported being vegetarian or vegan at the time of the dietary interview by sex and age of respondent and social class of the household reference person

Responding sample		Percentages
	Percentage reporting being vegetarian or vegan	Base
Sex and age of respondent		
Men aged (years):		
19–24	3	142
25–34	1	287
35–49	3	330
50–64	2	330
All men	2	1088
Women aged (years):		
19–24	12	136
25–34	11	275
35–49	5	415
50–64	4	337
All women	7	1163
Social class of household reference person		
Non-manual	6	1235
Manual	4	946
All*	5	2251

Note: *Includes those for whom a social class could not assigned.

Table 2.9

Types of foods avoided by respondents who said they were vegetarian or vegan

Those who said they were vegetarian or vegan	Percentages
Types of food avoided	All
Red meat	100
White meat	92
Fish	48
Eggs	21
Milk	5
Other dairy products (e.g. butter/cheese)	10
All animal products	29
Other	7
Base, number of vegetarian or vegan respondents*	*106*

Note: * Percentages add to more than 100 as some respondents reported avoiding more than one type of food.

Table 2.10(a)

Total quantities (grams) of food consumed in seven days by age of respondent: men consumers

Grams and percentages

Type of food	Men consumers aged (years):												All men		
	19–24			25–34			35–49			50–64					
	Mean	Median	% consumers	Mean	Median	% consumers	Mean	Median	% consumers	Mean	Median	% consumers	Mean	Median	% consumers
	g	g		g	g		g	g		g	g		g	g	
Pasta	425	337	66	463	376	58	382	330	52	356	284	42	406	332	52
Rice	394	334	54	476	300	59	418	300	58	373	300	46	420	300	54
Pizza	479	406	49	422	325	37	322	300	26	233	209	19	370	300	30
Other cereals	135	92	29	138	80	31	108	78	37	101	64	30	117	80	32
White bread	600	486	94	610	507	94	639	560	94	629	566	90	623	536	93
Wholemeal bread	*	*	19	450	380	29	376	289	36	363	320	40	381	308	33
Soft grain bread	*	*	3	*	*	1	*	*	2	*	*	5	*	*	3
Other bread	233	160	44	317	225	50	264	160	53	256	160	51	272	176	51
Whole grain & high fibre b'fast cereals	*	*	21	381	182	47	316	233	45	401	251	55	361	218	46
Other b'fast cereals	156	104	35	128	102	41	168	113	36	195	154	30	161	111	35
Biscuits	132	52	49	145	86	62	157	89	64	150	95	70	149	88	63
Fruit pies	*	*	5	138	110	14	*	*	12	184	122	20	165	113	14
Buns, cakes & pastries	193	158	50	200	140	53	246	196	60	295	207	65	246	177	58
Cereal-based milk puddings	*	*	11	*	*	11	224	142	18	252	200	21	248	200	16
Sponge-type puddings	*	*	6	*	*	5	*	*	5	*	*	8	165	110	6
Other cereal-based puddings	*	*	6	194	170	18	201	170	23	241	170	23	217	170	19
Whole milk	*	*	19	997	604	42	1190	767	36	996	601	38	1031	628	36
Semi-skimmed milk	983	718	77	1163	1048	78	1435	1250	76	1502	1345	68	1318	1102	74
Skimmed milk	*	*	5	*	*	12	910	689	17	1082	1004	19	1171	742	15
Cream	*	*	16	*	*	13	57	44	24	71	50	25	55	35	20
Other milk	*	*	12	434	300	17	*	*	9	*	*	10	492	300	12
Cottage cheese	-	-	-	*	*	2	*	*	3	*	*	4	*	*	3
Other cheese	150	125	63	147	98	79	144	124	79	145	115	82	146	112	78
Fromage frais	*	*	2	*	*	0	*	*	2	*	*	4	*	*	2
Yogurt	307	267	28	427	373	29	422	289	32	405	388	37	404	329	32
Other dairy desserts	*	*	5	*	*	5	*	*	10	*	*	9	144	115	8
Ice cream	*	*	17	179	129	23	151	120	32	176	139	29	166	122	27
Eggs	225	185	49	188	134	68	186	134	67	196	139	74	194	138	67
Egg dishes	*	*	10	*	*	11	145	120	14	188	143	21	185	140	15
Butter	66	35	37	38	30	38	66	48	42	83	58	40	64	40	40
Block margarine	*	*	1	-	-	-	*	*	0	*	*	0	*	*	0
Soft margarine, not polyunsaturated	39	40	31	26	20	40	32	20	30	33	18	28	31	20	32
Polyunsaturated margarine	*	*	5	*	*	3	*	*	3	*	*	3	*	*	3
Polyunsaturated oils	*	*	4	*	*	2	*	*	6	*	*	5	10	5	4
Other oils & cooking fats, not polyunsaturated	*	*	13	*	*	11	12	8	15	14	8	19	14	9	15
Polyunsaturated low fat spread	*	*	7	*	*	13	54	33	13	87	58	15	82	50	13
Other low fat spread	*	*	3	*	*	7	*	*	9	*	*	9	71	45	8
Polyunsaturated reduced fat spread	*	*	19	63	31	19	70	50	26	99	68	24	81	55	23
Other reduced fat spread	89	96	39	81	58	46	97	70	31	77	65	35	85	64	37
Bacon & ham	187	133	67	165	140	78	171	135	78	188	153	81	177	141	77
Beef, veal & dishes	483	404	66	431	310	70	441	371	68	423	342	66	438	347	68
Lamb & dishes	*	*	24	333	246	22	262	180	22	217	150	29	253	172	24
Pork & dishes	*	*	19	216	162	32	235	158	37	246	176	39	231	168	34
Coated chicken & turkey	222	164	39	201	181	31	216	198	26	181	163	13	207	170	25
Chicken & turkey dishes	436	361	80	501	423	81	526	439	79	386	280	86	463	369	82
Liver, liver products & dishes	*	*	5	*	*	10	143	84	13	139	105	15	133	100	12
Burgers & kebabs	295	223	66	292	244	44	232	179	32	*	*	11	261	205	33
Sausages	222	190	55	166	140	58	167	131	58	154	117	49	170	134	55
Meat pies & pastries	328	213	40	298	221	47	291	222	47	306	260	48	302	235	46
Other meat & meat products	135	114	28	187	92	26	184	125	32	212	128	36	189	120	31
Coated and/or fried white fish	202	180	31	203	177	30	195	170	38	203	172	43	200	175	36
Other white fish & dishes	*	*	14	*	*	9	194	148	16	299	210	26	244	171	17
Shellfish	*	*	8	105	64	15	122	77	23	148	80	19	135	80	18
Oily fish	*	*	18	195	148	33	215	150	45	194	141	54	198	140	41
Raw carrots	*	*	5	*	*	9	69	40	13	70	45	18	78	45	12
Other raw & salad vegetables	107	71	73	153	110	79	184	125	75	197	149	76	170	115	76
Raw tomatoes	97	79	56	157	121	61	159	105	66	180	146	77	159	119	67
Peas	117	92	42	130	84	53	152	103	62	172	125	67	150	103	59

Table 2.10(a) continued

Total quantities (grams) of food consumed in seven days by age of respondent: men consumers

Grams and percentages

Type of food	19–24			25–34			35–49			50–64			All men		
	Mean	Median	% consumers	Mean	Median	% consumers	Mean	Median	% consumers	Mean	Median	% consumers	Mean	Median	% consumers
	g	g		g	g		g	g		g	g		g	g	
Green beans	*	*	15	*	*	13	106	90	21	136	101	31	113	90	21
Baked beans	503	377	48	256	208	53	312	230	48	233	202	44	299	215	48
Leafy green vegetables	102	87	30	125	95	36	139	108	55	188	140	64	153	108	49
Carrots – not raw	81	80	50	104	84	49	112	90	57	119	98	67	109	88	57
Tomatoes – not raw	*	*	7	154	86	21	126	96	28	157	106	34	143	99	26
Vegetable dishes	*	*	23	350	173	32	436	301	26	267	218	27	335	200	28
Other vegetables	155	115	66	216	164	79	232	160	85	294	239	84	239	178	81
Potato chips	528	428	86	415	353	77	380	311	76	341	265	68	401	330	75
Other fried/roast potatoes & products	269	250	34	240	200	40	217	200	43	244	210	46	237	200	42
Potato products – not fried	*	*	8	*	*	9	*	*	6	*	*	8	167	160	8
Other potatoes & potato dishes	411	363	72	442	321	79	495	420	85	547	489	90	489	420	83
Savoury snacks	146	101	63	112	96	66	101	75	57	76	50	40	106	77	55
Apples & pears	251	237	31	393	328	40	444	364	55	498	383	59	437	351	49
Citrus fruits	*	*	10	265	200	20	350	277	29	292	218	31	299	225	25
Bananas	*	*	25	312	246	42	381	299	55	390	302	59	363	291	49
Canned fruit in juice	*	*	1	*	*	5	134	80	12	253	120	12	183	90	9
Canned fruit in syrup	*	*	4	*	*	0	*	*	7	*	*	9	236	195	6
Other fruit	*	*	8	285	167	28	258	155	43	354	255	52	303	185	37
Nuts & seeds	*	*	8	93	30	24	81	50	24	82	50	21	81	50	21
Table sugar	108	68	72	167	124	63	210	121	58	193	148	55	177	119	60
Preserves	*	*	18	45	34	26	69	43	38	93	60	49	74	45	36
Sweet spreads, fillings & icings	*	*	12	*	*	8	*	*	6	*	*	4	34	20	7
Sugar confectionery	*	*	20	49	28	21	77	34	24	64	42	15	73	41	20
Chocolate confectionery	171	106	62	138	96	61	131	93	58	108	82	42	134	92	54
Fruit juice	792	441	33	632	512	41	937	727	42	798	627	48	797	600	43
Concentrated soft drinks – not low calorie, as consumed	*	*	25	1852	1125	30	2067	1371	22	2076	1303	15	2144	1347	22
Carbonated soft drinks – not low calorie	2260	2230	92	1486	788	64	995	579	44	729	455	33	1389	730	52
Ready to drink soft drinks – not low calorie	*	*	24	480	378	14	*	*	11	*	*	9	545	375	13
Concentrated soft drinks – low calorie, as consumed	*	*	12	3041	2192	15	2514	1192	15	*	*	9	2616	1451	13
Carbonated soft drinks – low calorie	*	*	26	1854	999	30	1245	908	30	1109	628	22	1390	846	27
Ready to drink soft drinks – low calorie	-	-	-	*	*	0	*	*	1	*	*	1	*	*	1
Liqueurs	*	*	2	*	*	3	*	*	3	*	*	3	*	*	3
Spirits	*	*	21	*	*	11	242	83	21	214	109	25	197	92	19
Wine	*	*	19	784	650	30	899	633	43	1102	625	41	917	607	36
Fortified wine	*	*	3	*	*	3	*	*	4	*	*	8	293	131	5
Low alcohol & alcohol-free wine	-	-	-	-	-	-	*	*	1	*	*	0	*	*	0
Beer & lager	4164	2844	68	5049	3261	68	3760	2736	70	3937	2840	60	4213	2870	66
Low alcohol & alcohol-free beer & lager	-	-	-	*	*	4	*	*	4	*	*	4	*	*	3
Cider & perry	*	*	5	*	*	10	*	*	8	*	*	4	2741	1183	7
Low alcohol cider & perry	-	-	-	-	-	-	*	*	0	-	-	-	*	*	0
Alco-pops	*	*	16	*	*	5	*	*	2	-	-	-	1948	1116	4
Coffee, as consumed	4224	3077	56	5214	3129	76	6861	4940	74	5706	4317	75	5779	4267	72
Tea, as consumed	2083	1312	68	3010	2485	73	3847	3044	80	4862	3864	82	3766	3027	77
Herbal tea, as consumed	*	*	6	*	*	8	*	*	5	*	*	7	1033	548	6
Bottled water	*	*	15	1900	1190	25	1924	1110	25	1083	738	23	1656	1042	23
Tap water	1867	1229	53	2527	1336	56	2112	1223	58	2178	1040	64	2209	1197	59
Other beverages, dry weight	*	*	12	*	*	10	*	*	11	908	600	15	681	496	12
Soup	*	*	22	457	395	32	522	375	32	669	459	37	560	400	32
Savoury sauces, pickles, gravies & condiments	188	158	91	211	162	94	209	180	94	214	162	94	209	164	94
Base = number of respondents			108			219			253			253			833

Note: * Number of consumers is less than 30 and too small to calculate mean/median values reliably.

Table 2.10(b)

Total quantities (grams) of food consumed in seven days by age of respondent: women consumers

Grams and percentages

Type of food	Women consumers aged (years): 19–24 Mean	Median	% consumers	25–34 Mean	Median	% consumers	35–49 Mean	Median	% consumers	50–64 Mean	Median	% consumers	All women Mean	Median	% consumers
	g	g		g	g		g	g		g	g		g	g	
Pasta	417	408	64	333	288	60	338	265	50	266	212	46	330	261	53
Rice	241	200	51	342	236	58	371	268	53	303	200	42	332	228	51
Pizza	276	234	36	271	210	30	221	173	21	218	179	19	245	200	24
Other cereals	88	67	32	106	76	32	95	75	36	79	70	31	93	74	33
White bread	473	387	92	388	352	91	387	338	91	393	348	82	400	348	89
Wholemeal bread	*	*	15	249	198	35	238	182	43	236	197	47	236	192	39
Soft grain bread	*	*	1	*	*	1	*	*	1	*	*	4	*	*	2
Other bread	264	187	48	229	150	55	213	163	54	210	138	50	221	153	53
Whole grain & high fibre b'fast cereals	195	151	34	200	121	41	272	187	52	333	239	62	274	188	50
Other b'fast cereals	147	82	38	127	99	45	136	88	36	129	95	31	133	95	37
Biscuits	89	55	56	92	59	66	114	77	69	113	75	73	106	72	68
Fruit pies	*	*	3	*	*	9	*	*	9	146	110	17	137	110	11
Buns, cakes & pastries	144	127	34	180	151	63	179	137	65	221	156	67	190	145	62
Cereal-based milk puddings	*	*	12	*	*	7	205	151	16	219	192	20	210	162	15
Sponge-type puddings	*	*	1	*	*	4	*	*	5	*	*	4	163	117	4
Other cereal-based puddings	*	*	15	213	125	16	174	125	23	213	171	27	202	144	22
Whole milk	1128	640	32	755	519	43	958	592	34	763	555	32	866	555	35
Semi-skimmed milk	767	502	67	941	866	71	1150	966	74	1226	1132	74	1082	929	73
Skimmed milk	*	*	15	802	761	18	1255	1123	22	1290	1094	26	1179	1004	22
Cream	*	*	13	40	30	18	77	45	19	58	45	29	60	40	21
Other milk	*	*	17	*	*	11	522	318	12	415	130	14	409	282	13
Cottage cheese	*	*	6	*	*	10	*	*	5	*	*	9	172	141	8
Other cheese	125	92	63	116	92	78	110	91	71	109	83	77	113	90	73
Fromage frais	*	*	1	*	*	5	*	*	6	*	*	6	143	100	5
Yogurt	398	267	30	338	300	39	401	307	42	457	373	44	404	300	40
Other dairy desserts	*	*	10	*	*	11	135	102	10	*	*	10	130	104	10
Ice cream	*	*	28	144	120	26	136	113	26	145	120	31	145	114	28
Eggs	188	136	42	126	107	53	145	115	59	149	119	69	146	117	59
Egg dishes	*	*	7	143	110	15	152	121	17	170	146	19	158	137	16
Butter	30	18	35	38	24	39	44	27	43	59	40	47	46	27	42
Block margarine	-	-	-	*	*	1	-	-	-	*	*	1	*	*	0
Soft margarine, not polyunsaturated	*	*	22	22	14	25	26	18	23	26	14	22	24	14	23
Polyunsaturated margarine	*	*	1	*	*	1	*	*	2	*	*	3	*	*	2
Polyunsaturated oils	*	*	4	*	*	2	*	*	4	*	*	4	7	6	4
Other oils & cooking fats, not polyunsaturated	*	*	9	11	8	18	12	7	13	9	7	12	11	8	14
Polyunsaturated low fat spread	*	*	13	57	42	15	61	45	10	44	30	12	53	37	12
Other low fat spread	*	*	7	*	*	12	46	30	11	*	*	9	46	32	10
Polyunsaturated reduced fat spread	*	*	13	48	31	20	45	27	19	64	56	19	50	31	19
Other reduced fat spread	70	53	41	41	31	33	60	48	35	63	42	27	58	40	33
Bacon & ham	99	89	63	126	95	58	115	89	64	122	99	70	118	94	64
Beef, veal & dishes	456	362	51	327	300	54	535	291	61	351	300	59	426	300	58
Lamb & dishes	*	*	16	184	142	17	246	149	18	176	123	29	197	130	21
Pork & dishes	*	*	20	148	116	26	189	157	30	185	151	28	178	144	27
Coated chicken & turkey	229	167	34	171	154	26	179	164	26	168	153	14	183	164	24
Chicken & turkey dishes	329	306	80	375	330	73	409	309	74	305	256	81	360	300	77
Liver, liver products & dishes	*	*	4	*	*	3	*	*	8	*	*	10	97	80	7
Burgers & kebabs	307	205	34	232	204	22	178	162	18	*	*	8	216	177	18
Sausages	138	103	41	133	96	36	117	94	37	118	84	31	124	94	35
Meat pies & pastries	222	160	29	181	145	30	202	159	35	191	162	33	196	155	33
Other meat & meat products	*	*	22	*	*	13	123	83	20	153	107	29	129	85	21
Coated and/or fried white fish	*	*	24	141	150	30	171	155	32	168	155	41	162	152	33
Other white fish & dishes	*	*	10	*	*	11	229	183	18	232	178	28	220	181	18
Shellfish	*	*	16	131	76	20	144	85	23	181	100	21	151	90	21
Oily fish	176	128	38	167	122	37	180	124	48	217	156	58	190	133	47
Raw carrots	*	*	12	48	33	17	68	49	19	57	40	15	62	40	16
Other raw & salad vegetables	141	101	72	188	115	84	214	153	82	203	148	80	197	136	81
Raw tomatoes	131	77	57	155	113	69	179	146	69	181	150	79	170	136	70
Peas	125	70	37	99	77	47	117	77	55	115	90	58	113	80	52

NDNS adults aged 19 to 64, Volume 1 2002

Table 2.10(b) continued

Total quantities (grams) of food consumed in seven days by age of respondent: women consumers

Grams and percentages

Type of food	Women consumers aged (years):												All women		
	19–24			25–34			35–49			50–64					
	Mean	Median	% consumers	Mean	Median	% consumers	Mean	Median	% consumers	Mean	Median	% consumers	Mean	Median	% consumers
	g	g		g	g		g	g		g	g		g	g	
Green beans	*	*	20	98	87	15	99	85	19	114	90	33	103	86	22
Baked beans	198	167	45	225	194	46	205	168	41	192	155	35	206	167	41
Leafy green vegetables	96	68	43	123	86	45	148	105	56	181	150	70	150	107	56
Carrots – not raw	83	60	42	91	61	45	100	88	58	117	80	68	103	80	56
Tomatoes – not raw	*	*	10	136	101	24	125	85	22	96	70	28	118	85	23
Vegetable dishes	338	197	30	439	287	41	461	290	32	317	208	27	406	259	33
Other vegetables	131	110	75	212	159	78	214	175	82	243	194	82	213	162	80
Potato chips	434	350	76	302	241	72	271	227	66	247	202	62	294	233	67
Other fried/roast potatoes & products	166	150	43	155	121	39	179	150	42	179	150	44	172	150	42
Potato products – not fried	*	*	8	*	*	4	*	*	5	*	*	4	115	82	5
Other potatoes & potato dishes	455	363	78	415	354	77	431	365	87	494	417	88	449	375	84
Savoury snacks	108	88	76	92	75	69	73	54	57	51	35	39	80	60	57
Apples & pears	283	259	40	365	272	50	348	250	54	482	312	61	390	291	54
Citrus fruits	*	*	22	301	192	22	326	203	31	363	209	40	327	200	30
Bananas	291	300	28	300	259	52	344	259	56	379	304	69	344	277	56
Canned fruit in juice	*	*	3	*	*	7	*	*	7	176	134	14	169	117	8
Canned fruit in syrup	*	*	2	*	*	3	*	*	4	*	*	10	165	121	5
Other fruit	306	186	41	256	151	40	362	208	52	502	353	63	387	216	51
Nuts & seeds	*	*	17	54	26	19	69	31	19	58	28	23	62	32	20
Table sugar	90	69	45	103	53	50	129	70	48	118	40	47	115	54	48
Preserves	*	*	21	60	42	36	52	34	41	57	39	45	55	36	39
Sweet spreads, fillings & icings	*	*	11	*	*	7	*	*	8	*	*	5	29	20	7
Sugar confectionery	61	46	31	49	31	24	54	30	27	89	45	21	63	35	25
Chocolate confectionery	118	77	60	111	83	58	106	72	62	94	59	50	106	71	57
Fruit juice	701	454	50	625	437	50	690	456	44	766	566	47	697	500	47
Concentrated soft drinks – not low calorie, as consumed	1892	1032	38	1725	846	23	1152	724	20	1473	980	14	1516	841	21
Carbonated soft drinks – not low calorie	1848	1151	64	895	614	47	853	513	38	706	332	32	1012	568	42
Ready to drink soft drinks – not low calorie	*	*	20	601	514	15	727	552	13	*	*	11	644	500	14
Concentrated soft drinks – low calorie, as consumed	*	*	27	2311	1133	19	*	*	9	*	*	8	1885	1028	13
Carbonated soft drinks – low calorie	2305	1240	35	1806	1152	50	1271	754	34	1066	580	26	1521	885	36
Ready to drink soft drinks – low calorie	*	*	4	*	*	2	*	*	3	*	*	2	*	*	2
Liqueurs	*	*	10	*	*	8	*	*	8	*	*	6	72	50	8
Spirits	*	*	27	116	73	18	139	69	19	162	92	23	139	88	21
Wine	636	479	37	710	610	45	752	611	46	842	625	49	759	600	45
Fortified wine	*	*	3	*	*	6	*	*	9	*	*	11	216	125	8
Low alcohol & alcohol-free wine	*	*	1	*	*	1	*	*	0	*	*	0	*	*	1
Beer & lager	2593	1421	34	1654	1150	33	1658	1019	25	1153	574	13	1731	1136	24
Low alcohol & alcohol-free beer & lager	-	-	-	*	*	2	*	*	1	*	*	3	*	*	2
Cider & perry	*	*	2	*	*	3	*	*	3	*	*	4	*	*	3
Alco-pops	*	*	21	*	*	12	*	*	6	*	*	2	1258	825	8
Coffee, as consumed	3988	3052	50	3703	2882	60	5152	3271	75	4841	3050	81	4659	3049	70
Tea, as consumed	2094	1631	69	3092	2422	76	4067	3442	78	4434	3885	80	3745	3136	77
Herbal tea, as consumed	*	*	4	*	*	11	1392	972	15	1567	1113	14	1348	1024	12
Bottled water	*	*	21	1675	747	32	1778	1013	24	1281	662	30	1566	943	27
Tap water	2059	1335	71	2449	1399	77	2346	1537	72	2630	1628	72	2420	1430	73
Other beverages, dry weight	*	*	10	452	342	20	626	455	19	654	461	21	569	399	19
Soup	*	*	25	493	441	32	495	385	34	515	393	44	490	400	35
Savoury sauces, pickles, gravies & condiments	151	131	91	174	131	89	187	150	92	158	115	93	171	132	91
Base = number of respondents			104			210			318			259			891

Note: * Number of consumers is less than 30 and too small to calculate mean/median values reliably.

27

Table 2.10(c)

Main differences in the eating behaviour of respondents by sex and age group

Foods more likely to be eaten by:

All men (compared with women)	Men aged 19–24 years [1]	Men aged 50–64 years [2]
white bread*	pasta*	wholemeal bread*
eggs*	pizza**	whole grain & high fibre breakfast cereals**
soft margarine not pufa**	coated chicken & turkey**	fruit pies**
bacon & ham**	burgers & kebabs**	other cereal-based puddings**
beef, veal & dishes**	potato chips*	whole milk*
pork & dishes*	savoury snacks*	skimmed milk**
liver, liver products & dishes*	carbonated soft drinks nlc**	cottage cheese*
burgers & kebabs**	alco-pops*	eggs*
sausages**		pork & dishes*
meat pies & pastries**		liver, liver products & dishes*
other meat & meat products**		oily fish**
baked beans*		raw carrots*
potato chips*		peas*
table sugar**		green beans*
carbonated soft drinks nlc**		leafy green vegetables**
beer & lager**		tomatoes – not raw**
cider & perry*		other potatoes and potato dishes*
		apples & pears**
		citrus fruits**
		bananas**
		canned fruit in juice**
		other fruit**
		preserves**
		wine*
		low alcohol and alcohol-free beer & lager*
		coffee*

All women (compared with men)	Women aged 19–24 years [1]	Women aged 50–64 years [2]
skimmed milk*	coated chicken & turkey*	wholemeal bread**
cottage cheese**	burgers & kebabs**	whole grain & high fibre breakfast cereals**
fromage frais*	savoury snacks**	fruit pies**
yogurt*	carbonated soft drinks nlc**	buns, cakes & pastries**
other fruit**	concentrated soft drinks nlc**	cream*
carbonated soft drinks lc*	concentrated soft drinks lc*	eggs**
liqueurs**	beer & lager*	egg dishes*
wine**	alco-pops**	coated and/or fried white fish*
alco-pops*		other white fish & dishes**
herbal tea**		oily fish*
tap water**		raw tomatoes*
other beverages*		peas*
		leafy green vegetables**
		carrots – not raw**
		tomatoes – not raw**
		apples & pears*
		citrus fruits*
		bananas**
		canned fruit in juice*
		canned fruit in syrup*
		other fruit*
		preserves**
		fortified wine*
		low alcohol and alcohol-free beer & lager*
		coffee**
		herbal tea*
		soup*

Note: [1] Compared with same sex aged 50 to 64 years
       [2] Compared with same sex aged 19 to 24 years
       * $p<0.05$
       ** $p<0.01$
       pufa: polyunsaturated
       nlc: not low calorie
       lc: low calorie

Table 2.11(a)

Total quantities (grams) of food consumed in seven days by age of respondent: men, including non-consumers

Grams

Type of food	All men aged (years):								All men	
	19–24		25–34		35–49		50–64			
	Mean	sd	Mean	sd	Mean	sd*	Mean	sd	Mean	sd
	g	g	g	g	g	g	g	g	g	g
Pasta	280	325	266	346	198	275	151	241	212	297
Rice	211	271	280	454	243	405	171	321	226	382
Pizza	236	315	154	283	84	171	45	107	110	224
Other cereals	39	93	43	118	40	81	30	75	38	92
White bread	565	410	570	435	604	440	566	459	578	441
Wholemeal bread	54	129	131	294	136	262	146	241	127	253
Soft grain bread	5	31	1	10	3	25	35	212	12	119
Other bread	103	167	160	235	140	247	132	233	138	231
Whole grain & high fibre b'fast cereals	54	161	177	691	144	230	223	391	165	440
Other b'fast cereals	54	113	52	87	61	117	58	120	57	110
Biscuits	65	137	90	135	101	177	104	156	95	156
Fruit pies	6	28	20	62	20	65	37	97	23	73
Buns, cakes & pastries	97	139	106	156	147	205	191	263	143	209
Cereal-based milk puddings	34	110	28	110	40	121	53	132	40	120
Sponge-type puddings	7	25	8	36	8	46	15	71	10	51
Other cereal-based puddings	18	91	35	87	46	103	56	130	42	108
Whole milk	130	333	421	929	426	1161	384	802	373	923
Semi-skimmed milk	755	1007	902	960	1095	1142	1015	1193	976	1100
Skimmed milk	48	306	218	1269	150	502	206	599	172	789
Cream	3	7	5	17	14	36	18	44	11	33
Other milk	55	172	76	367	44	225	61	520	59	370
Cottage cheese	-	-	3	26	5	45	7	55	4	41
Other cheese	94	126	116	162	114	110	120	132	114	134
Fromage frais	5	40	1	8	4	32	5	34	4	30
Yogurt	85	181	123	242	136	362	149	258	130	283
Other dairy desserts	6	28	7	29	13	48	16	66	11	48
Ice cream	27	77	42	103	49	92	52	110	45	99
Eggs	109	156	128	158	125	144	145	159	130	154
Egg dishes	20	73	25	102	20	61	40	97	27	87
Butter	24	76	14	27	28	52	34	67	26	56
Block margarine	1	5	-	-	0	6	0	1	0	4
Soft margarine, not polyunsaturated	12	21	11	19	9	27	9	28	10	25
Polyunsaturated margarine	3	14	1	8	2	17	1	5	1	12
Polyunsaturated oils	0	1	0	3	1	3	1	5	0	4
Other oils & cooking fats, not polyunsaturated	3	13	1	5	2	7	3	10	2	8
Polyunsaturated low fat spread	8	44	13	50	7	27	13	43	11	41
Other low fat spread	1	8	5	29	5	22	9	40	6	29
Polyunsaturated reduced fat spread	19	44	12	45	19	43	24	66	18	52
Other reduced fat spread	34	58	37	72	30	69	27	51	31	64
Bacon & ham	125	139	128	128	133	139	153	153	137	141
Beef, veal & dishes	315	334	302	376	299	352	281	335	296	351
Lamb & dishes	45	95	73	203	58	150	62	139	61	157
Pork & dishes	39	94	69	132	87	167	95	195	79	161
Coated chicken & turkey	85	158	62	110	58	117	24	70	52	112
Chicken & turkey dishes	345	335	405	458	419	408	334	361	380	401
Liver, liver products & dishes	3	23	12	46	18	68	21	64	15	58
Burgers & kebabs	192	224	128	217	73	194	15	61	86	187
Sausages	121	174	96	125	98	124	75	117	93	130
Meat pies & pastries	131	227	139	207	137	215	148	217	140	215
Other meat & meat products	37	73	49	167	58	127	78	203	59	160
Coated and/or fried white fish	63	109	61	114	74	116	86	122	73	117
Other white fish & dishes	24	74	19	74	31	91	77	183	41	124
Shellfish	20	80	15	51	28	80	28	93	24	78
Oily fish	23	66	64	134	97	185	105	158	81	155
Raw carrots	5	33	9	33	9	36	13	40	10	36
Other raw & salad vegetables	78	100	121	166	137	180	150	189	129	172
Raw tomatoes	55	70	96	152	106	146	138	149	106	143
Peas	49	81	70	106	94	128	115	145	88	125

Table 2.11(a) continued

Total quantities (grams) of food consumed in seven days by age of respondent: men, including non-consumers

Grams

Type of food	All men aged (years):								All men	
	19–24		25–34		35–49		50–64			
	Mean	sd	Mean	sd	Mean	sd	Mean	sd	Mean	sd
	g	g	g	g	g	g	g	g	g	g
Green beans	11	27	11	33	22	54	42	93	24	63
Baked beans	241	390	135	188	150	230	104	163	144	234
Leafy green vegetables	30	57	46	83	76	103	121	141	76	112
Carrots – not raw	40	47	51	68	63	91	79	86	62	80
Tomatoes – not raw	6	28	32	109	36	85	54	166	37	118
Vegetable dishes	48	108	112	287	116	337	72	177	93	260
Other vegetables	101	124	171	191	196	231	247	233	193	215
Potato chips	455	355	319	312	289	286	233	271	302	306
Other fried/roast potatoes & products	92	146	95	141	94	138	111	157	99	146
Potato products – not fried	22	79	12	46	10	46	11	48	13	52
Other potatoes & potato dishes	295	271	351	349	418	360	494	370	407	356
Savoury snacks	92	124	75	85	58	93	31	55	58	89
Apples & pears	76	139	158	277	242	368	296	435	215	355
Citrus fruits	14	45	53	146	103	234	91	201	75	189
Bananas	71	163	129	215	210	308	229	313	176	278
Canned fruit in juice	2	19	7	41	16	72	30	154	16	97
Canned fruit in syrup	8	50	2	28	13	69	24	107	13	74
Other fruit	19	78	79	234	110	232	185	320	113	256
Nuts and seeds	1	5	22	69	20	58	17	62	17	59
Table sugar	77	103	105	174	122	221	105	166	107	181
Preserves	12	33	12	27	26	59	46	79	26	59
Sweet spreads, fillings & icings	2	8	5	26	1	6	1	9	2	15
Sugar confectionery	26	92	10	30	19	55	10	33	15	51
Chocolate confectionery	107	174	84	116	76	111	45	80	73	116
Fruit juice	264	685	258	481	397	755	385	624	340	644
Concentrated soft drinks – not low calorie, as consumed	782	2389	550	1261	447	1450	315	1141	477	1485
Carbonated soft drinks – not low calorie	2063	1963	946	1437	441	875	243	584	725	1309
Ready to drink soft drinks – not low calorie	163	403	65	205	50	220	50	216	69	249
Concentrated soft drinks – low calorie, as consumed	349	1471	461	1507	380	1415	174	762	335	1292
Carbonated soft drinks – low calorie	325	879	557	1671	376	985	242	793	376	1153
Ready to drink soft drinks – low calorie	-	-	2	27	4	38	10	127	5	74
Liqueurs	1	3	4	40	3	21	4	38	3	31
Spirits	16	38	19	74	50	166	52	178	38	141
Wine	101	276	236	516	385	706	454	986	330	735
Fortified wine	10	78	7	61	17	172	20	118	14	122
Low alcohol & alcohol-free wine	-	-	-	-	5	68	1	10	2	38
Beer & lager	2806	3565	3451	4467	2637	3467	2357	3639	2788	3833
Low alcohol & alcohol-free beer & lager	-	-	37	205	110	1184	24	162	51	667
Cider & perry	238	2555	188	788	303	1780	71	408	194	1422
Low alcohol cider & perry	-	-	-	-	6	128	-	-	2	70
Alco-pops	450	1304	52	266	14	131	-	-	76	514
Coffee, as consumed	2326	3953	3958	5551	5038	6447	4321	5283	4184	5640
Tea, as consumed	1404	1743	2185	2408	3094	3014	3979	3739	2904	3112
Herbal tea, as consumed	40	183	46	184	36	222	122	655	65	399
Bottled water	276	903	463	1315	478	1379	243	612	377	1122
Tap water	988	1742	1409	2857	1239	2246	1383	2616	1295	2479
Other beverages, dry weight	124	532	43	170	52	184	134	442	84	339
Soup	123	250	143	256	165	376	249	503	179	384
Savoury sauces, pickles, gravies & condiments	171	137	199	198	196	157	202	187	195	176
Base = number of respondents		108		219		253		253		833

Table 2.11(b)

Total quantities (grams) of food consumed in seven days by age of respondent: women, including non-consumers

Grams

Type of food	All women aged (years):								All women	
	19–24		25–34		35–49		50–64			
	Mean	sd	Mean	sd	Mean	sd	Mean	sd	Mean	sd
	g	g	g	g	g	g	g	g	g	g
Pasta	270	270	198	248	169	246	123	222	174	246
Rice	123	174	199	293	196	327	127	237	168	282
Pizza	100	171	81	168	46	115	42	104	59	135
Other cereals	28	63	34	75	34	82	25	49	31	70
White bread	438	531	353	253	353	272	323	295	354	317
Wholemeal bread	24	72	88	166	102	171	110	170	92	163
Soft grain bread	1	9	3	39	2	19	6	37	3	30
Other bread	127	219	126	191	116	164	106	177	117	181
Whole grain & high fibre b'fast cereals	66	133	82	189	142	245	205	298	137	245
Other b'fast cereals	56	111	56	96	49	104	40	84	49	98
Biscuits	50	82	61	81	79	105	82	98	72	96
Fruit pies	3	19	10	39	13	45	24	72	14	52
Buns, cakes & pastries	49	93	114	131	117	140	148	180	117	149
Cereal-based milk puddings	19	57	16	87	33	100	44	114	30	98
Sponge-type puddings	2	21	9	61	9	48	5	25	7	44
Other cereal-based puddings	41	197	35	128	41	90	60	120	44	125
Whole milk	353	1035	322	625	326	810	242	546	304	733
Semi-skimmed milk	516	652	670	776	850	990	906	1066	785	941
Skimmed milk	198	681	145	397	282	667	340	766	257	651
Cream	7	36	7	20	15	54	17	39	13	42
Other milk	56	143	30	129	61	366	60	312	53	287
Cottage cheese	9	40	16	62	11	57	15	62	13	58
Other cheese	78	118	90	93	78	79	84	84	83	89
Fromage frais	2	18	7	44	9	43	8	47	7	42
Yogurt	119	250	131	211	168	279	201	328	163	278
Other dairy desserts	12	42	14	51	13	53	13	46	13	49
Ice cream	48	120	38	83	35	80	46	90	40	89
Eggs	79	133	67	91	87	112	103	113	86	111
Egg dishes	12	49	21	64	26	77	32	84	25	74
Butter	10	20	15	31	19	34	27	48	19	37
Block margarine	-	-	0	1	0	0	0	2	0	1
Soft margarine, not polyunsaturated	5	13	5	17	6	14	6	21	6	17
Polyunsaturated margarine	0	2	0	3	2	18	1	11	1	12
Polyunsaturated oils	0	2	0	1	0	2	0	2	0	2
Other oils & cooking fats, not polyunsaturated	1	5	2	6	2	7	1	4	1	6
Polyunsaturated low fat spread	5	20	9	31	6	25	5	18	6	24
Other low fat spread	1	2	6	20	5	22	5	22	5	20
Polyunsaturated reduced fat spread	3	9	10	28	9	27	12	34	9	28
Other reduced fat spread	29	56	14	27	21	43	17	42	19	41
Bacon & ham	62	71	73	100	74	94	86	93	76	93
Beef, veal & dishes	232	305	175	230	326	2112	208	273	245	1279
Lamb & dishes	25	75	30	86	44	158	50	110	40	122
Pork & dishes	35	95	39	88	57	121	52	101	48	105
Coated chicken & turkey	78	142	44	92	48	97	24	74	43	98
Chicken & turkey dishes	264	235	273	290	304	351	249	232	276	293
Liver, liver products & dishes	3	15	4	27	7	32	10	36	6	31
Burgers & kebabs	104	264	50	127	32	85	11	43	39	126
Sausages	56	94	48	89	43	73	37	81	44	82
Meat pies & pastries	65	129	55	113	71	150	63	113	64	129
Other meat & meat products	22	73	14	58	25	72	44	105	27	81
Coated and/or fried white fish	37	79	41	75	56	95	69	96	54	90
Other white fish & dishes	18	66	21	65	40	121	65	136	40	111
Shellfish	22	67	26	86	33	91	38	145	31	106
Oily fish	68	152	63	114	86	152	126	180	90	155
Raw carrots	11	45	8	30	12	40	8	28	10	35
Other raw & salad vegetables	102	132	158	203	176	197	162	182	159	189
Raw tomatoes	74	118	106	139	124	149	143	151	120	145
Peas	46	147	46	74	64	99	68	86	59	97

Table 2.11(b) continued

Total quantities (grams) of food consumed in seven days by age of respondent: women, including non-consumers

Grams

Type of food	All women aged (years):								All women	
	19–24		25–34		35–49		50–64			
	Mean	sd	Mean	sd	Mean	sd	Mean	sd	Mean	sd
	g	g	g	g	g	g	g	g	g	g
Green beans	16	40	14	45	19	49	37	77	23	58
Baked beans	89	154	103	154	84	145	68	121	84	142
Leafy green vegetables	41	67	55	91	82	113	126	143	84	117
Carrots – not raw	35	57	41	68	58	69	79	96	57	78
Tomatoes – not raw	13	47	33	80	28	75	27	63	27	70
Vegetable dishes	101	246	182	357	147	349	87	244	132	314
Other vegetables	98	99	166	191	176	189	199	202	171	187
Potato chips	327	326	217	248	180	201	152	176	198	230
Other fried/roast potatoes & products	72	97	60	104	76	123	78	117	72	114
Potato products – not fried	9	37	2	14	4	23	7	43	5	31
Other potatoes & potato dishes	353	360	320	298	375	306	433	345	376	325
Savoury snacks	83	80	64	73	41	56	20	34	45	62
Apples & pears	113	173	183	280	188	290	294	447	209	337
Citrus fruits	47	113	66	177	100	229	146	297	99	233
Bananas	81	165	156	228	194	278	260	295	191	267
Canned fruit in juice	4	27	9	79	12	96	24	80	14	82
Canned fruit in syrup	6	45	3	18	5	33	19	71	8	47
Other fruit	127	295	103	233	188	344	318	479	198	372
Nuts and seeds	11	56	10	34	14	48	13	41	12	44
Table sugar	41	83	51	107	63	162	56	135	55	135
Preserves	8	21	22	44	21	39	26	45	21	41
Sweet spreads, fillings & icings	3	10	2	7	3	17	1	8	2	12
Sugar confectionery	19	42	12	37	14	41	19	106	16	66
Chocolate confectionery	70	124	65	89	65	96	47	81	60	94
Fruit juice	353	527	316	492	302	558	358	619	327	558
Concentrated soft drinks – not low calorie, as consumed	734	1714	393	1139	236	685	199	903	320	1038
Carbonated soft drinks – not low calorie	1194	1648	421	719	321	735	230	649	420	913
Ready to drink soft drinks – not low calorie	102	245	92	265	95	351	72	292	88	303
Concentrated soft drinks – low calorie, as consumed	307	691	439	1661	180	1117	167	853	252	1171
Carbonated soft drinks – low calorie	800	2196	892	1652	433	1003	281	849	540	1352
Ready to drink soft drinks – low calorie	8	43	10	80	11	81	4	31	8	66
Liqueurs	6	28	7	29	6	30	3	16	5	26
Spirits	32	82	20	66	27	99	37	113	29	95
Wine	234	425	318	547	347	569	410	682	345	587
Fortified wine	4	30	16	157	18	103	22	87	17	109
Low alcohol & alcohol-free wine	5	44	8	74	2	32	2	36	4	47
Beer & lager	864	1935	549	1193	407	1240	145	587	418	1210
Low alcohol & alcohol-free beer & lager	-	-	6	50	6	59	18	160	9	96
Cider & perry	69	535	49	336	65	820	19	123	48	551
Alco-pops	337	953	95	330	82	403	22	270	97	467
Coffee, as consumed	1980	3551	2234	3305	3887	5469	3933	5903	3287	5047
Tea, as consumed	1438	1865	2331	2658	3164	3348	3546	3258	2876	3098
Herbal tea, as consumed	24	150	108	402	208	798	222	780	167	669
Bottled water	316	785	537	1608	433	1276	385	960	430	1238
Tap water	1471	2025	1885	2647	1688	2328	1900	2989	1771	2581
Other beverages, dry weight	28	89	88	248	119	354	137	407	106	330
Soup	89	215	159	290	166	313	227	386	173	324
Savoury sauces, pickles, gravies & condiments	138	114	155	142	172	165	147	138	157	147
Base = number of respondents		104		210		318		259		891

Table 2.11(c)

Main differences in the total quantity of foods consumed by men and women, including non-consumers

Greater quantity eaten by:

All men	All women
rice*	cottage cheese*
pizza**	other raw & salad vegetables*
white bread**	other fruit**
wholemeal bread*	herbal tea**
biscuits*	tap water**
semi-skimmed milk*	
other cheese**	
eggs**	
soft margarine, not pufa**	
pufa reduced fat spread**	
other reduced fat spread**	
bacon & ham**	
lamb & dishes*	
pork & dishes**	
chicken & turkey dishes**	
liver, liver products & dishes*	
burgers & kebabs**	
sausages**	
meat pies & pastries**	
other meat & meat products**	
coated and/or fried white fish*	
peas**	
baked beans**	
potato chips**	
other fried/roast potatoes & products**	
potato products – not fried*	
savoury snacks*	
table sugar**	
carbonated soft drinks nlc**	
beer & lager**	
coffee*	
savoury sauces, pickles, gravies & condiments**	

Greater quantity eaten by men aged (compared with women in same age group):

19–24 years	25–34 years	35–49 years	50–64 years
pizza*	white bread**	pizza*	white bread**
bacon & ham*	eggs**	white bread**	other cheese*
beer & lager*	other reduced fat spread**	semi-skimmed milk*	eggs*
	bacon & ham**	other cheese**	bacon & ham**
	beef, veal & dishes*	eggs*	pork & dishes*
	chicken & turkey dishes*	pufa reduced fat spread*	chicken & turkey dishes*
	burgers & kebabs**	bacon & ham**	sausages**
	sausages**	chicken & turkey dishes**	meat pies & pastries**
	meat pies & pastries**	burgers & kebabs*	peas**
	potato chips*	sausages**	potato chips**
	table sugar*	meat pies & pastries**	table sugar*
	carbonated soft drinks nlc**	other meat & meat products**	preserves*
	beer & lager**	peas*	beer & lager**
	coffee*	baked beans**	savoury sauces, pickles, gravies & condiments*
		potato chips**	
		table sugar**	
		beer & lager**	

Greater quantity eaten by women aged (compared with men in same age group):

19–24 years	25–34 years	35–49 years	50–64 years
other fruit*		skimmed milk*	other fruit*
		other fruit*	
		alco-pops*	
		herbal teas**	
		other beverages*	

Note: * p<0.05
      ** p<0.01
      nlc: not low calorie
      pufa: polyunsaturated

Table 2.12(a)

Total quantities (grams) of food consumed in seven days by region: men consumers

Grams and percentages

Type of food	Region											
	Scotland			Northern			Central, South West and Wales			London and the South East		
	Mean	Median	% consumers	Mean	Median	% consumers	Mean	Median	% consumers	Mean	Median	% consumers
	g	g		g	g		g	g		g	g	
Pasta	466	447	66	343	298	42	415	340	51	423	337	59
Rice	462	311	57	359	300	52	387	322	47	488	300	63
Pizza	*	*	29	362	303	32	401	299	29	339	300	30
Other cereals	*	*	18	134	80	39	112	79	28	113	80	35
White bread	562	503	94	680	617	95	658	574	93	538	470	90
Wholemeal bread	*	*	35	384	320	33	439	383	33	309	212	34
Soft grain bread	*	*	6	*	*	3	*	*	2	*	*	3
Other bread	313	212	48	242	160	42	273	176	47	281	177	65
Whole grain & high fibre b'fast cereals	317	252	52	287	195	38	394	222	47	392	245	50
Other b'fast cereals	168	151	46	167	133	38	155	100	36	160	115	28
Biscuits	153	86	62	118	72	65	172	100	65	151	93	61
Fruit pies	*	*	12	132	111	14	171	116	14	188	125	14
Buns, cakes & pastries	180	117	55	236	139	52	278	222	62	230	169	60
Cereal-based milk puddings	*	*	22	227	173	13	276	214	20	236	200	13
Sponge-type puddings	*	*	3	*	*	3	*	*	7	*	*	8
Other cereal-based puddings	*	*	22	226	173	19	232	174	20	212	159	19
Whole milk	*	*	40	1103	776	37	1002	554	37	807	361	33
Semi-skimmed milk	1574	1403	75	1252	1051	70	1302	1089	77	1328	1022	74
Skimmed milk	*	*	14	1054	732	21	1675	1149	13	*	*	11
Cream	*	*	25	61	40	15	45	30	20	67	45	24
Other milk	*	*	2	*	*	10	412	330	14	406	297	14
Cottage cheese	*	*	3	*	*	2	*	*	2	*	*	4
Other cheese	143	111	77	144	106	74	144	118	77	150	107	84
Fromage frais	*	*	2	*	*	2	*	*	3	*	*	2
Yogurt	*	*	32	496	375	34	334	270	29	374	318	34
Other dairy desserts	*	*	8	*	*	7	*	*	8	*	*	8
Ice cream	*	*	26	143	120	19	172	125	30	174	129	31
Eggs	206	149	66	162	123	67	207	160	71	204	135	63
Egg dishes	*	*	17	165	155	14	204	140	16	178	122	13
Butter	*	*	32	68	48	29	80	47	40	53	36	53
Block margarine	-	-	-	*	*	0	*	*	1	-	-	-
Soft margarine, not polyunsaturated	*	*	28	36	21	36	34	20	28	25	21	35
Polyunsaturated margarine	*	*	3	*	*	3	*	*	3	*	*	3
Polyunsaturated oils	*	*	2	*	*	3	*	*	4	*	*	6
Other oils & cooking fats, not polyunsaturated	*	*	9	*	*	11	16	10	15	16	9	20
Polyunsaturated low fat spread	*	*	14	102	47	17	77	59	12	*	*	10
Other low fat spread	*	*	18	*	*	8	*	*	7	*	*	6
Polyunsaturated reduced fat spread	*	*	30	82	63	29	86	76	17	67	52	22
Other reduced fat spread	*	*	29	76	57	37	103	77	42	65	52	33
Bacon & ham	191	164	77	187	155	84	180	147	76	156	124	73
Beef, veal & dishes	418	380	80	452	350	74	440	316	63	428	350	65
Lamb & dishes	*	*	17	250	149	20	241	153	22	272	181	33
Pork & dishes	*	*	23	197	150	35	215	169	39	263	183	30
Coated chicken & turkey	*	*	29	227	200	24	183	158	24	212	167	27
Chicken & turkey dishes	515	370	85	429	350	82	456	351	83	493	406	80
Liver, liver products & dishes	*	*	11	112	100	13	113	80	10	*	*	12
Burgers & kebabs	*	*	32	199	194	30	259	205	35	314	230	33
Sausages	215	172	54	170	123	57	153	120	56	180	150	51
Meat pies & pastries	263	209	54	325	274	56	312	246	46	265	200	35
Other meat & meat products	182	118	46	220	114	33	191	117	28	155	128	29
Coated and/or fried white fish	*	*	44	225	170	32	187	180	41	194	180	32
Other white fish & dishes	*	*	18	197	166	14	242	170	15	229	203	22
Shellfish	*	*	12	109	79	16	176	121	16	120	71	23
Oily fish	*	*	38	206	130	42	192	140	37	199	164	45
Raw carrots	*	*	11	*	*	12	80	64	12	53	39	13
Other raw & salad vegetables	166	106	72	165	105	73	154	112	77	192	141	80
Raw tomatoes	166	128	58	166	115	69	155	119	66	155	122	67
Peas	131	125	55	169	110	57	158	120	63	126	89	56

Table 2.12(a) continued

Total quantities (grams) of food consumed in seven days by region: men consumers

Grams and percentages

Type of food	Region											
	Scotland			Northern			Central, South West and Wales			London and the South East		
	Mean	Median	% consumers	Mean	Median	% consumers	Mean	Median	% consumers	Mean	Median	% consumers
	g	g		g	g		g	g		g	g	
Green beans	*	*	12	89	75	16	121	90	22	121	90	26
Baked beans	203	142	48	299	230	51	324	227	50	291	200	44
Leafy green vegetables	*	*	38	148	106	47	139	106	50	166	120	54
Carrots – not raw	110	89	47	107	88	58	110	86	63	110	86	50
Tomatoes – not raw	*	*	31	123	91	26	131	109	25	137	86	24
Vegetable dishes	*	*	17	320	185	24	259	140	22	398	265	41
Other vegetables	249	177	80	205	159	81	230	180	78	280	208	84
Potato chips	447	397	80	393	309	76	445	364	81	327	233	66
Other fried/roast potatoes & products	*	*	26	224	200	34	240	203	45	247	220	50
Potato products – not fried	*	*	15	*	*	6	*	*	8	*	*	7
Other potatoes & potato dishes	543	517	86	493	409	87	487	388	81	473	426	83
Savoury snacks	*	*	40	103	76	54	100	80	62	119	81	53
Apples & pears	513	417	54	425	366	46	398	320	49	473	357	51
Citrus fruits	*	*	35	295	230	24	327	198	21	284	233	28
Bananas	336	280	54	352	292	48	378	289	45	365	294	53
Canned fruit in juice	*	*	6	*	*	11	*	*	10	*	*	5
Canned fruit in syrup	*	*	11	*	*	6	*	*	5	*	*	4
Other fruit	*	*	40	249	169	32	283	191	34	332	219	45
Nuts and seeds	*	*	9	67	54	16	92	47	21	73	30	29
Table sugar	183	82	46	198	149	56	193	139	66	136	85	60
Preserves	*	*	31	85	48	34	69	47	36	64	43	38
Sweet spreads, fillings & icings	*	*	3	*	*	5	*	*	8	*	*	8
Sugar confectionery	*	*	15	65	33	23	67	40	15	79	42	25
Chocolate confectionery	102	82	46	124	86	57	145	98	55	136	92	53
Fruit juice	706	512	46	828	749	35	712	507	40	879	600	52
Concentrated soft drinks – not low calorie, as consumed	*	*	9	2649	1461	18	2091	1310	31	1913	1251	19
Carbonated soft drinks – not low calorie	1564	750	55	1406	834	47	1421	712	54	1288	660	55
Ready to drink soft drinks – not low calorie	*	*	8	*	*	10	558	375	13	568	320	17
Concentrated soft drinks – low calorie, as consumed	*	*	14	*	*	11	2300	1485	15	2939	1721	12
Carbonated soft drinks – low calorie	*	*	37	1741	791	25	1321	883	27	1203	828	26
Ready to drink soft drinks – low calorie	*	*	2	*	*	1	*	*	1	*	*	1
Liqueurs	*	*	2	*	*	3	*	*	3	*	*	3
Spirits	*	*	23	204	75	15	182	90	21	136	81	20
Wine	*	*	32	861	614	32	713	500	32	1119	650	45
Fortified wine	*	*	5	*	*	2	*	*	4	*	*	9
Low alcohol & alcohol-free wine	-	-	-	*	*	1	*	*	1	-	-	-
Beer & lager	3812	3763	68	4820	3259	71	4095	2837	64	3812	2296	64
Low alcohol & alcohol-free beer & lager	*	*	3	*	*	3	*	*	4	*	*	4
Cider & perry	*	*	2	*	*	9	*	*	10	*	*	4
Low alcohol cider & perry	-	-	-	*	*	0	-	-	-	-	-	-
Alco-pops	*	*	2	*	*	3	*	*	4	*	*	5
Coffee, as consumed	6221	4301	74	7031	5295	70	5369	4200	72	5000	3209	75
Tea, as consumed	3086	2712	68	4014	3328	74	4049	3280	84	3301	2802	74
Herbal tea, as consumed	*	*	5	*	*	3	*	*	5	*	*	12
Bottled water	*	*	12	1690	1437	16	1365	1000	19	1888	1191	36
Tap water	2481	1653	80	1796	1031	51	2411	1343	53	2235	1210	67
Other beverages, dry weight	*	*	11	*	*	9	704	602	13	633	424	15
Soup	732	565	51	496	383	27	499	393	29	600	485	36
Savoury sauces, pickles, gravies & condiments	140	122	94	197	164	93	221	183	95	222	178	93
Base = number of respondents			65			234			294			240

Note: * Number of consumers is less than 30 and too small to calculate mean/median values reliably.

Table 2.12(b)

Total quantities (grams) of food consumed in seven days by region: women consumers

Grams and percentages

Type of food	Region											
	Scotland			Northern			Central, South West and Wales			London and the South East		
	Mean	Median	% consumers	Mean	Median	% consumers	Mean	Median	% consumers	Mean	Median	% consumers
	g	g		g	g		g	g		g	g	
Pasta	385	297	61	334	266	51	311	250	52	333	260	54
Rice	296	258	52	275	200	45	289	218	50	424	265	56
Pizza	*	*	33	250	189	24	218	187	20	250	220	28
Other cereals	*	*	9	98	80	37	77	72	39	115	70	30
White bread	364	337	91	411	351	90	400	361	88	398	323	87
Wholemeal bread	*	*	36	215	182	43	246	183	37	245	204	38
Soft grain bread	*	*	5	*	*	3	*	*	2	*	*	1
Other bread	181	122	47	206	143	55	243	160	53	218	160	53
Whole grain & high fibre b'fast cereals	316	166	47	250	181	52	257	174	50	307	209	48
Other b'fast cereals	109	91	47	136	96	35	142	82	36	127	107	37
Biscuits	104	82	64	99	63	66	108	78	69	110	73	69
Fruit pies	*	*	8	*	*	13	156	133	9	124	102	11
Buns, cakes & pastries	150	128	65	187	142	55	198	156	63	193	135	66
Cereal-based milk puddings	*	*	15	229	190	15	188	145	14	229	198	14
Sponge-type puddings	*	*	3	*	*	4	*	*	4	*	*	5
Other cereal-based puddings	*	*	24	179	125	22	220	164	22	181	130	22
Whole milk	*	*	41	869	687	37	821	558	33	970	470	35
Semi-skimmed milk	1209	1033	71	1104	1022	73	1072	876	76	1045	924	69
Skimmed milk	*	*	12	1123	1003	26	1235	1085	24	1165	906	17
Cream	*	*	14	70	33	17	55	45	23	65	40	23
Other milk	*	*	14	347	174	13	325	281	11	546	305	15
Cottage cheese	*	*	8	*	*	10	*	*	8	*	*	5
Other cheese	126	115	74	109	79	69	114	100	74	110	85	76
Fromage frais	*	*	6	*	*	5	*	*	6	*	*	3
Yogurt	*	*	38	456	440	42	385	296	39	381	260	40
Other dairy desserts	*	*	11	*	*	9	*	*	9	117	96	13
Ice cream	*	*	24	134	116	25	158	120	29	138	104	29
Eggs	137	111	50	140	119	62	141	111	59	159	128	58
Egg dishes	*	*	18	166	154	14	142	119	15	158	119	18
Butter	48	27	45	46	28	39	44	24	45	48	30	41
Block margarine	*	*	3	-	-	-	*	*	0	*	*	0
Soft margarine, not polyunsaturated	*	*	27	36	24	23	20	14	22	21	15	23
Polyunsaturated margarine	*	*	2	*	*	2	*	*	4	*	*	1
Polyunsaturated oils	*	*	5	*	*	2	*	*	3	*	*	5
Other oils & cooking fats, not polyunsaturated	*	*	18	*	*	10	9	9	13	13	9	16
Polyunsaturated low fat spread	*	*	14	50	35	17	41	31	9	68	57	12
Other low fat spread	*	*	14	*	*	13	41	34	10	*	*	7
Polyunsaturated reduced fat spread	*	*	14	63	37	17	44	28	18	45	29	21
Other reduced fat spread	*	*	23	50	34	28	64	56	39	56	37	33
Bacon & ham	116	77	54	121	96	69	108	89	68	128	95	59
Beef, veal & dishes	1415	349	54	341	299	61	364	301	59	343	290	53
Lamb & dishes	*	*	9	177	121	20	177	132	20	234	138	25
Pork & dishes	*	*	20	183	154	22	168	142	32	188	120	28
Coated chicken & turkey	*	*	35	158	138	24	193	167	24	192	165	19
Chicken & turkey dishes	376	288	77	337	285	76	366	320	80	367	270	73
Liver, liver products & dishes	*	*	5	*	*	7	*	*	7	*	*	7
Burgers & kebabs	*	*	15	167	122	19	248	194	20	208	202	15
Sausages	*	*	33	117	87	37	119	97	38	131	94	31
Meat pies & pastries	*	*	35	194	158	39	190	155	31	217	161	29
Other meat & meat products	*	*	24	116	80	24	130	79	20	117	73	19
Coated and/or fried white fish	*	*	29	163	148	40	164	150	35	163	165	27
Other white fish & dishes	*	*	26	194	178	18	210	170	17	252	170	18
Shellfish	*	*	18	157	100	18	131	70	22	175	91	23
Oily fish	*	*	44	192	140	44	145	100	46	241	164	53
Raw carrots	*	*	8	60	30	16	58	30	15	68	46	20
Other raw & salad vegetables	144	97	83	203	141	77	188	128	79	214	146	85
Raw tomatoes	170	138	70	166	137	66	150	119	70	194	153	75
Peas	*	*	33	116	78	57	124	97	58	95	68	45

NDNS adults aged 19 to 64, Volume 1 2002

Table 2.12(b) continued

Total quantities (grams) of food consumed in seven days by region: women consumers

Grams and percentages

Type of food	Region											
	Scotland			Northern			Central, South West and Wales			London and the South East		
	Mean	Median	% consumers	Mean	Median	% consumers	Mean	Median	% consumers	Mean	Median	% consumers
	g	g		g	g		g	g		g	g	
Green beans	*	*	17	108	90	14	107	90	22	95	66	31
Baked beans	*	*	32	213	174	44	213	168	43	193	154	37
Leafy green vegetables	134	95	48	150	105	53	144	103	57	162	125	58
Carrots – not raw	*	*	41	104	85	57	103	78	62	104	80	51
Tomatoes – not raw	*	*	26	98	78	21	129	85	22	116	85	24
Vegetable dishes	*	*	24	293	161	26	352	233	31	534	334	42
Other vegetables	225	173	71	205	158	79	206	152	82	225	180	82
Potato chips	262	210	64	319	253	72	317	256	70	242	200	61
Other fried/roast potatoes & products	*	*	27	151	120	34	168	150	46	191	162	48
Potato products – not fried	*	*	6	*	*	5	*	*	4	*	*	5
Other potatoes & potato dishes	454	465	86	429	361	87	468	396	85	442	354	79
Savoury snacks	76	53	58	79	57	55	76	60	58	86	74	55
Apples & pears	451	256	52	432	300	45	363	281	55	381	302	59
Citrus fruits	*	*	38	360	233	29	266	161	31	368	228	29
Bananas	315	218	64	344	255	52	345	292	53	351	292	58
Canned fruit in juice	*	*	21	*	*	7	210	123	9	*	*	6
Canned fruit in syrup	*	*	11	*	*	5	*	*	5	*	*	4
Other fruit	379	279	59	432	213	43	379	201	50	370	211	58
Nuts and seeds	*	*	12	46	33	14	53	28	20	78	44	28
Table sugar	*	*	42	115	54	55	143	59	46	89	51	47
Preserves	*	*	42	60	40	32	55	36	42	50	33	40
Sweet spreads, fillings & icings	*	*	5	*	*	5	*	*	7	*	*	9
Sugar confectionery	*	*	24	67	45	20	69	30	27	55	34	27
Chocolate confectionery	106	72	73	116	77	51	104	60	60	99	80	56
Fruit juice	910	683	53	598	482	44	703	441	45	708	526	50
Concentrated soft drinks – not low calorie, as consumed	*	*	24	1243	806	19	1640	934	23	1665	871	20
Carbonated soft drinks – not low calorie	*	*	39	1012	568	45	1129	599	41	878	601	40
Ready to drink soft drinks - not low calorie	*	*	18	*	*	12	679	501	16	*	*	11
Concentrated soft drinks – low calorie, as consumed	*	*	11	1623	1133	15	1339	823	13	2237	1120	14
Carbonated soft drinks – low calorie	1665	1184	45	1536	965	33	1432	744	37	1580	713	33
Ready to drink soft drinks – low calorie	-	-	-	*	*	3	*	*	2	*	*	3
Liqueurs	*	*	17	*	*	5	*	*	8	*	*	7
Spirits	*	*	29	152	100	19	132	69	20	136	75	22
Wine	989	726	45	808	750	39	688	507	47	757	559	49
Fortified wine	*	*	15	*	*	4	*	*	7	*	*	10
Low alcohol & alcohol-free wine	-	-	-	*	*	2	*	*	1	-	-	-
Beer & lager	*	*	14	2103	1435	33	1600	1099	23	1472	764	20
Low alcohol & alcohol-free beer & lager	-	-	-	*	*	3	*	*	1	*	*	2
Cider & perry	*	*	5	*	*	3	*	*	4	*	*	1
Alco-pops	*	*	5	*	*	6	995	660	10	*	*	7
Coffee, as consumed	4426	3100	71	5688	3467	74	4598	3040	70	3843	2446	68
Tea, as consumed	3534	3315	74	3991	3509	76	4033	3367	78	3233	2820	77
Herbal tea, as consumed	*	*	12	*	*	5	1814	1462	13	1086	685	18
Bottled water	*	*	26	1525	1116	23	1372	755	24	1793	837	35
Tap water	1877	1264	79	2212	1211	70	2271	1362	71	2882	2007	78
Other beverages, dry weight	*	*	12	529	263	13	518	402	20	657	428	23
Soup	606	516	70	524	400	38	427	394	30	463	300	31
Savoury sauces, pickles, gravies & condiments	123	92	88	186	143	95	176	134	94	164	127	87
Base = number of respondents			66			229			327			268

Note: * Number of consumers is less than 30 and too small to calculate mean/median values reliably.

Table 2.12(c)

Main differences in the eating behaviour of respondents by sex and region – summary table

Food type and sub-group	Men		Women	
	Less likely to eat in:	Compared with:	Less likely to eat in:	Compared with:
Cereals and cereal products				
pasta	N	Sc*, L & SE*		
rice	CSW & W	L & SE*		
other bread	N, CSW & W	L & SE**		
other cereals	Sc	N*	Sc	N**, CSW & W**, L & SE**
Milk, milk products, eggs & egg dishes				
skimmed milk	L & SE	N*		
other milk	Sc	N*, CSW & W**, L & SE**		
ice cream	N	L & SE*		
Fats				
butter	N	L & SE**		
	CSW & W	L & SE*		
other reduced fat spread			Sc, N	CSW & W*
Meat and meat products				
lamb & dishes	N	L & SE*	Sc	L & SE*
meat pies & pastries	L & SE	N**		
Fish & fish dishes				
coated &/or fried white fish			L & SE	N*
Vegetables				
carrots – raw			Sc	L & SE*
peas			Sc	N*, CSW & W**
			L & SE	CSW & W*
green beans			N	L & SE**
carrots – not raw	L & SE	CSW & W*	Sc	CSW & W*
vegetable dishes	Sc, N, CSW & W	L & SE**	Sc	L & SE*
			N	L & SE**
potato chips	L & SE	CSW & W**		
other fried & roast potatoes & products	Sc, N	L & SE*	Sc	CSW & W*, L & SE*
			N	L & SE*
savoury snacks	Sc	CSW & W*		
Fruit & nuts				
apples & pears			N	L & SE*
canned fruit in juice			L & SE	Sc*
other fruit			N	L & SE*
nuts & seeds	Sc	L & SE**	Sc	L & SE*
	N	L & SE*	N	L & SE**
Sugars, preserves & confectionery				
sugar confectionery	CSW & W	L & SE*		
chocolate confectionery			N, L & SE	Sc*
Beverages				
fruit juice	N	L & SE*		
concentrated soft drinks nlc	Sc	CSW & W**		
	N, L & SE	CSW & W*		
ready-to-drink soft drinks lc			Sc	L & SE*
beer & lager			Sc, L & SE	N*
cider & perry	Sc	CSW & W*		
wine	CSW & W	L & SE*		
fortified wine	N	L & SE*		
herbal tea, as consumed	N, CSW & W	L & SE*	N	CSW & W*, L & SE**
tap water	N	Sc**, L & SE*		
	CSW & W	Sc**, L & SE*		
bottled water	Sc, N, CSW & W	L & SE**	N, CSW & W	L & SE*
Miscellaneous				
soup	N	Sc*	N, CSW & W, L & SE	Sc**
savoury sauces, pickles, gravies & condiments			L & SE	N*, CSW & W*

Note: Sc: Scotland   N: Northern   CSW & W: Central, South West and Wales   L & SE: London and the South East
* p<0.05
** p<0.01
pufa: polyunsaturated
nlc: not low calorie
lc: low calorie

Table 2.13(a)

Total quantities (grams) of food consumed in seven days by whether someone in respondent's household was receiving certain benefits: men consumers

Grams and percentages

Type of food	Whether receiving benefits						
	Receiving benefits				Not receiving benefits		
	Mean	Median	% consumers		Mean	Median	% consumers
	g	g			g	g	
Pasta	455	323	44		400	333	54
Rice	513	310	50		407	300	55
Pizza	*	*	19		379	300	31
Other cereals	88	80	28		121	80	33
White bread	706	632	94		610	522	93
Wholemeal bread	*	*	23		373	305	35
Soft grain bread	-	-	-		*	*	3
Other bread	218	148	32		277	178	54
Whole grain & high fibre b'fast cereals	338	259	30		363	210	48
Other b'fast cereals	154	105	33		162	118	36
Biscuits	145	96	59		150	87	64
Fruit pies	*	*	13		172	117	14
Buns, cakes & pastries	186	136	52		254	184	59
Cereal-based milk puddings	*	*	14		247	200	17
Sponge-type puddings	*	*	3		167	110	7
Other cereal-based puddings	*	*	15		216	170	20
Whole milk	1251	864	48		985	591	34
Semi-skimmed milk	1036	822	64		1354	1148	76
Skimmed milk	*	*	12		1166	747	15
Cream	*	*	9		55	34	22
Other milk	*	*	14		530	300	12
Cottage cheese	-	-	-		*	*	3
Other cheese	139	97	69		147	116	80
Fromage frais	*	*	2		*	*	2
Yogurt	*	*	18		414	350	34
Other dairy desserts	*	*	5		150	118	8
Ice cream	*	*	21		167	120	28
Eggs	222	138	70		189	139	67
Egg dishes	*	*	7		189	140	16
Butter	71	36	32		63	40	41
Block margarine	*	*	1		*	*	0
Soft margarine, not polyunsaturated	35	20	27		31	20	33
Polyunsaturated margarine	*	*	2		*	*	3
Polyunsaturated oils	*	*	5		11	5	4
Other oils & cooking fats, not polyunsaturated	*	*	13		14	8	15
Polyunsaturated low fat spread	*	*	11		81	50	13
Other low fat spread	*	*	7		75	51	8
Polyunsaturated reduced fat spread	*	*	22		82	55	23
Other reduced fat spread	88	54	45		84	66	36
Bacon & ham	197	166	65		174	138	79
Beef, veal & dishes	453	333	67		436	350	68
Lamb & dishes	*	*	17		242	175	25
Pork & dishes	*	*	26		234	168	35
Coated chicken & turkey	*	*	26		202	170	25
Chicken & turkey dishes	498	441	65		459	361	84
Liver, liver products & dishes	*	*	8		133	100	12
Burgers & kebabs	340	206	35		248	204	33
Sausages	172	152	58		170	129	54
Meat pies & pastries	310	237	54		300	235	45
Other meat & meat products	177	105	39		191	125	30
Coated and/or fried white fish	225	170	46		195	180	35
Other white fish & dishes	*	*	14		243	170	17
Shellfish	*	*	6		134	80	19
Oily fish	*	*	26		200	140	43
Raw carrots	*	*	10		76	49	13
Other raw & salad vegetables	148	100	58		172	119	79
Raw tomatoes	154	95	58		160	121	68
Peas	192	143	61		144	100	59

Table 2.13(a) continued

Total quantities (grams) of food consumed in seven days by whether someone in respondent's household was receiving certain benefits: men consumers

Grams and percentages

Type of food	Whether receiving benefits					
	Receiving benefits			Not receiving benefits		
	Mean	Median	% consumers	Mean	Median	% consumers
	g	g		g	g	
Green beans	*	*	15	113	90	22
Baked beans	293	211	51	300	217	48
Leafy green vegetables	145	104	35	154	109	52
Carrots – not raw	113	85	52	109	88	58
Tomatoes – not raw	*	*	25	139	89	26
Vegetable dishes	*	*	16	327	200	29
Other vegetables	218	156	71	242	181	82
Potato chips	479	450	83	387	324	74
Other fried/roast potatoes & products	214	192	32	240	200	43
Potato products – not fried	*	*	5	162	160	8
Other potatoes & potato dishes	523	447	75	485	413	84
Savoury snacks	122	82	45	104	75	57
Apples & pears	455	386	31	436	345	52
Citrus fruits	*	*	16	301	206	26
Bananas	348	271	32	364	292	51
Canned fruit in juice	*	*	14	158	88	8
Canned fruit in syrup	*	*	10	239	176	5
Other fruit	*	*	15	304	185	41
Nuts & seeds	*	*	10	77	48	23
Table sugar	206	153	74	172	108	58
Preserves	72	41	30	75	47	36
Sweet spreads, fillings & icings	*	*	2	35	27	7
Sugar confectionery	*	*	20	71	35	20
Chocolate confectionery	159	98	50	130	91	55
Fruit juice	681	721	28	808	596	45
Concentrated soft drinks – not low calorie, as consumed	*	*	26	2166	1303	22
Carbonated soft drinks – not low calorie	1680	876	58	1339	704	51
Ready to drink soft drinks – not low calorie	*	*	7	548	375	13
Concentrated soft drinks – low calorie, as consumed	*	*	16	2923	1829	12
Carbonated soft drinks – low calorie	*	*	25	1421	754	27
Ready-to-drink soft drinks – low calorie	*	*	1	*	*	1
Liqueurs	*	*	3	*	*	3
Spirits	*	*	13	198	92	20
Wine	*	*	15	935	625	39
Fortified wine	*	*	1	299	132	5
Low alcohol & alcohol-free wine	*	*	1	*	*	0
Beer & lager	3576	2290	45	4275	2969	69
Low alcohol & alcohol-free beer & lager	*	*	3	*	*	3
Cider & perry	*	*	7	2502	1151	7
Low alcohol cider & perry	-	-	-	*	*	0
Alco-pops	*	*	1	1948	1107	4
Coffee, as consumed	7428	5322	66	5554	4203	73
Tea, as consumed	3588	3229	75	3793	3021	77
Herbal tea, as consumed	*	*	2	1057	581	7
Bottled water	*	*	8	1600	1000	25
Tap water	2205	1130	45	2210	1200	61
Other beverages, dry weight	*	*	8	683	500	13
Soup	561	400	28	560	402	33
Savoury sauces, pickles, gravies & condiments	160	117	87	215	177	94
Base = number of respondents			110			723

Note: * Number of consumers is less than 30 and too small to calculate mean/median values reliably.

Table 2.13(b)

Total quantities (grams) of food consumed in seven days by whether someone in respondent's household was receiving certain benefits: women consumers

Grams and percentages

Type of food	Whether receiving benefits					
	Receiving benefits			Not receiving benefits		
	Mean	Median	% consumers	Mean	Median	% consumers
	g	g		g	g	
Pasta	358	304	39	326	253	56
Rice	359	228	47	327	229	51
Pizza	311	231	22	233	188	25
Other cereals	84	80	31	94	70	34
White bread	402	359	93	399	342	88
Wholemeal bread	258	220	22	234	188	43
Soft grain bread	-	-	-	*	*	3
Other bread	227	159	38	221	153	56
Whole grain & high fibre b'fast cereals	197	141	36	285	192	53
Other b'fast cereals	150	115	37	130	92	37
Biscuits	111	78	57	106	70	70
Fruit pies	*	*	8	140	110	11
Buns, cakes & pastries	173	133	49	193	147	64
Cereal-based milk puddings	*	*	12	212	159	15
Sponge-type puddings	*	*	3	169	117	4
Other cereal-based puddings	*	*	11	204	142	24
Whole milk	1086	869	49	797	460	32
Semi-skimmed milk	998	755	64	1097	944	74
Skimmed milk	*	*	14	1212	1011	23
Cream	*	*	8	62	40	24
Other milk	*	*	11	411	248	13
Cottage cheese	*	*	3	167	141	8
Other cheese	105	80	62	114	93	76
Fromage frais	*	*	3	145	100	6
Yogurt	293	203	25	418	310	43
Other dairy desserts	*	*	8	137	106	11
Ice cream	*	*	19	147	112	29
Eggs	134	120	54	148	116	60
Egg dishes	*	*	11	148	120	17
Butter	40	22	26	47	29	45
Block margarine	*	*	1	*	*	0
Soft margarine, not polyunsaturated	*	*	18	23	14	24
Polyunsaturated margarine	*	*	5	*	*	2
Polyunsaturated oils	*	*	4	*	*	4
Other oils & cooking fats, not polyunsaturated	*	*	7	11	8	15
Polyunsaturated low fat spread	*	*	11	51	37	12
Other low fat spread	*	*	11	49	39	10
Polyunsaturated reduced fat spread	*	*	18	51	29	18
Other reduced fat spread	57	40	35	58	40	33
Bacon & ham	105	87	61	120	94	65
Beef, veal & dishes	372	340	53	436	300	58
Lamb & dishes	*	*	19	173	128	21
Pork & dishes	148	120	23	183	146	28
Coated chicken & turkey	194	167	25	181	159	23
Chicken & turkey dishes	371	271	73	357	305	77
Liver, liver products & dishes	*	*	4	95	80	7
Burgers & kebabs	211	195	27	217	166	16
Sausages	120	103	43	125	90	34
Meat pies & pastries	223	161	44	189	150	30
Other meat & meat products	185	115	22	118	80	21
Coated and/or fried white fish	162	152	33	162	152	33
Other white fish & dishes	*	*	15	217	178	19
Shellfish	*	*	13	146	91	23
Oily fish	164	127	27	193	133	51
Raw carrots	*	*	9	63	40	18
Other raw & salad vegetables	136	84	66	206	144	84
Raw tomatoes	118	86	50	177	144	75
Peas	122	89	48	112	79	53

Table 2.13(b) continued

Total quantities (grams) of food consumed in seven days by whether someone in respondent's household was receiving certain benefits: women consumers

Grams and percentages

Type of food	Whether receiving benefits						
	Receiving benefits				Not receiving benefits		
	Mean	Median	% consumers		Mean	Median	% consumers
	g	g			g	g	
Green beans	*	*	11		101	84	25
Baked beans	230	182	39		202	167	41
Leafy green vegetables	159	124	40		149	105	59
Carrots – not raw	95	73	46		104	80	58
Tomatoes – not raw	*	*	17		116	85	24
Vegetable dishes	509	287	20		394	257	35
Other vegetables	175	145	69		220	171	82
Potato chips	370	300	75		276	210	66
Other fried/roast potatoes & products	178	154	33		171	150	44
Potato products – not fried	*	*	4		113	88	5
Other potatoes & potato dishes	385	348	75		461	385	85
Savoury snacks	85	63	61		78	60	56
Apples & pears	359	201	42		395	308	56
Citrus fruits	*	*	19		337	213	33
Bananas	279	239	39		352	279	59
Canned fruit in juice	*	*	7		173	120	9
Canned fruit in syrup	*	*	5		170	122	5
Other fruit	414	159	25		385	217	57
Nuts & seeds	*	*	14		57	30	21
Table sugar	186	102	58		97	45	46
Preserves	40	24	21		56	37	42
Sweet spreads, fillings & icings	*	*	5		28	20	7
Sugar confectionery	*	*	16		64	35	27
Chocolate confectionery	115	70	49		104	71	59
Fruit juice	851	548	39		672	478	49
Concentrated soft drinks – not low calorie, as consumed	1421	608	20		1534	894	21
Carbonated soft drinks – not low calorie	1336	810	49		931	524	40
Ready to drink soft drinks – not low calorie	*	*	10		669	501	14
Concentrated soft drinks – low calorie, as consumed	*	*	12		1979	1022	14
Carbonated soft drinks – low calorie	1238	902	25		1559	883	38
Ready-to-drink soft drinks – low calorie	*	*	3		*	*	2
Liqueurs	*	*	5		67	50	8
Spirits	134	90	20		140	78	21
Wine	687	495	20		765	606	51
Fortified wine	*	*	7		186	116	8
Low alcohol & alcohol-free wine	*	*	1		*	*	1
Beer & lager	2299	1435	27		1603	1045	24
Low alcohol & alcohol-free beer & lager	*	*	1		*	*	2
Cider & perry	*	*	4		*	*	3
Alco-pops	*	*	11		1100	660	7
Coffee, as consumed	6231	3895	65		4369	2882	72
Tea, as consumed	3856	2486	70		3725	3234	78
Herbal tea, as consumed	*	*	7		1381	1032	13
Bottled water	*	*	14		1602	976	30
Tap water	2123	1192	64		2472	1587	75
Other beverages, dry weight	*	*	11		565	385	20
Soup	424	294	29		501	400	36
Savoury sauces, pickles, gravies & condiments	146	112	88		176	135	92
Base = number of respondents			150				741

Note: * Number of consumers is less than 30 and too small to calculate mean/median values reliably.

Table 2.13(c)

Main differences in the eating behaviour of respondents by household receipt of benefits – summary table

Foods less likely to be eaten by:	Households in receipt of benefits (compared with those not receiving)
Men	soft grain bread**
	other bread**
	whole grain & high fibre breakfast cereals*
	cream**
	cottage cheese**
	yogurt*
	chicken & turkey dishes**
	shellfish**
	oily fish*
	other raw & salad vegetables**
	leafy green vegetables*
	vegetable dishes*
	apples & pears**
	bananas**
	other fruit**
	nuts & seeds*
	sweet spreads, fillings & icings*
	fruit juice*
	wine**
	fortified wine*
	beer & lager**
	herbal teas*
	bottled water**
	tap water*
Women	pasta**
	wholemeal bread**
	soft grain bread**
	other bread**
	whole grain & high fibre breakfast cereals**
	biscuits*
	buns, cakes & pastries**
	other cereal-based puddings**
	skimmed milk*
	cream**
	cottage cheese*
	other cheese*
	yogurt**
	ice-cream*
	butter**
	other oils & cooking fats not pufa*
	shellfish*
	oily fish**
	raw carrots*
	other raw & salad vegetables**
	raw tomatoes**
	green beans**
	leafy green vegetables**
	carrots – not raw*
	vegetable dishes**
	other vegetables*
	other fried/roast potatoes or products*
	other potatoes & potato dishes*
	apples & pears*
	citrus fruits**
	bananas**
	other fruit**
	preserves**
	sugar confectionery*
	carbonated soft drinks lc*
	wine**
	bottled water**
	tap water*
	other beverages*

Foods more likely to be eaten by:	Households in receipt of benefits (compared with those not receiving)
Men	table sugar*
Women	whole milk**
	burgers & kebabs*
	meat pies & pastries*
	table sugar*

Note: * p<0.05
       ** p<0.01
       pufa: polyunsaturated
       nlc: not low calorie   lc: low calorie

Table 2.14

Total quantities (grams) of food consumed in seven days: consumers and all respondents

Grams and percentages

Type of food	Consumers			All, including non-consumers	
	Mean	Median	% consumers	Mean	sd
	g	g		g	g
Pasta	366	295	53	193	272
Rice	376	273	52	196	335
Pizza	312	236	27	84	185
Other cereals	104	80	33	34	82
White bread	510	421	91	462	398
Wholemeal bread	300	226	36	109	212
Soft grain bread	298	114	3	8	86
Other bread	245	160	52	127	207
Whole grain & high fibre b'fast cereals	314	198	48	151	353
Other b'fast cereals	146	103	36	53	104
Biscuits	126	78	66	83	129
Fruit pies	153	110	12	19	63
Buns, cakes & pastries	216	155	60	130	181
Cereal-based milk puddings	229	185	15	35	109
Sponge-type puddings	164	110	5	8	47
Other cereal-based puddings	209	168	21	43	117
Whole milk	947	602	36	337	831
Semi-skimmed milk	1198	1011	73	877	1025
Skimmed milk	1176	944	18	215	722
Cream	58	37	21	12	38
Other milk	447	289	12	56	329
Cottage cheese	168	121	5	9	51
Other cheese	129	100	76	98	114
Fromage frais	150	110	4	6	37
Yogurt	404	319	36	147	281
Other dairy desserts	136	107	9	12	49
Ice cream	155	120	27	42	94
Eggs	170	125	63	107	135
Egg dishes	170	140	15	26	80
Butter	54	35	41	22	47
Block margarine	*	*	0	0	3
Soft margarine, not polyunsaturated	28	19	27	8	21
Polyunsaturated margarine	46	25	3	1	12
Polyunsaturated oils	9	5	4	0	3
Other oils and cooking fats, not polyunsaturated	13	8	14	2	7
Polyunsaturated low fat spread	67	42	13	8	34
Other low fat spread	56	39	9	5	25
Polyunsaturated reduced fat spread	66	42	21	14	42
Other reduced fat spread	72	51	35	25	54
Bacon & ham	149	117	71	105	122
Beef, veal & dishes	432	320	62	270	951
Lamb & dishes	226	150	22	51	140
Pork & dishes	207	153	30	63	136
Coated chicken & turkey	195	167	24	48	105
Chicken & turkey dishes	411	329	79	326	353
Liver, liver products & dishes	119	86	9	11	46
Burgers & kebabs	244	204	25	61	160
Sausages	151	117	45	68	111
Meat pies & pastries	256	202	39	101	180
Other meat & meat products	164	110	26	43	126
Coated and/or fried white fish	181	170	35	63	104
Other white fish & dishes	231	176	18	40	118
Shellfish	144	81	19	28	94
Oily fish	194	137	44	86	155
Raw carrots	69	44	14	10	36
Other raw & salad vegetables	184	125	78	144	181
Raw tomatoes	165	128	69	113	144
Peas	132	94	55	73	113

Table 2.14 continued

Total quantities (grams) of food consumed in seven days: consumers and all respondents

Grams and percentages

Type of food	Consumers			All, including non-consumers	
	Mean	Median	% consumers	Mean	sd
	g	g		g	g
Green beans	108	90	22	23	60
Baked beans	255	199	44	113	194
Leafy green vegetables	152	108	53	80	115
Carrots – not raw	106	85	56	59	79
Tomatoes – not raw	131	85	24	32	97
Vegetable dishes	374	233	30	113	290
Other vegetables	226	170	80	182	202
Potato chips	348	270	71	248	274
Other fried/roast potatoes & products	203	175	42	85	131
Potato products – not fried	146	120	6	9	42
Other potatoes & potato dishes	469	396	84	391	341
Savoury snacks	92	72	56	52	77
Apples & pears	412	316	51	212	346
Citrus fruits	315	203	28	87	213
Bananas	352	283	52	184	272
Canned fruit in juice	176	107	8	15	89
Canned fruit in syrup	201	141	5	11	62
Other fruit	353	204	44	157	324
Nuts & seeds	71	41	20	15	52
Table sugar	149	86	54	80	161
Preserves	64	40	37	24	50
Sweet spreads, fillings & icings	32	20	7	2	13
Sugar confectionery	67	37	23	15	59
Chocolate confectionery	119	81	56	66	106
Fruit juice	743	548	45	333	601
Concentrated soft drinks – not low calorie, as consumed	1828	1080	22	396	1276
Carbonated soft drinks – not low calorie	1215	660	47	567	1132
Ready to drink soft drinks – not low calorie	598	404	13	79	278
Concentrated soft drinks – low calorie, as consumed	2230	1150	13	292	1231
Carbonated soft drinks – low calorie	1466	848	31	461	1262
Ready to drink soft drinks – low calorie	379	302	2	6	70
Liqueurs	82	50	5	4	29
Spirits	166	90	20	34	119
Wine	826	605	41	338	662
Fortified wine	244	125	6	16	116
Low alcohol & alcohol-free wine	*	*	1	3	43
Beer & lager	3516	2260	44	1563	3043
Low alcohol & alcohol-free beer & lager	1148	574	3	29	469
Cider & perry	2336	1141	5	119	1067
Low alcohol cider & perry	*	*	0	1	49
Alco-pops	1480	990	6	87	490
Coffee, as consumed	5208	3460	71	3720	5359
Tea, as consumed	3755	3074	77	2889	3104
Herbal tea, as consumed	1246	893	9	118	558
Bottled water	1606	1000	25	404	1183
Tap water	2330	1344	66	1541	2543
Other beverages, dry weight	612	420	16	95	335
Soup	522	400	34	176	354
Savoury sauces, pickles, gravies & condiments	190	150	92	175	163
Base = number of respondents			1724		

Note: * Number of consumers is less than 30 and too small to calculate mean/median values reliably.

Table 2.15(a)

Proportion of respondents consuming portions of fruit and vegetables, including composite dishes*, by number of portions consumed and sex and age of respondent: fruit and vegetables (all fruit juice counted as one portion; all baked beans and other pulses counted as one portion)

Cumulative percentages

Average daily number of portions of fruit and vegetables consumed	Men aged (years):				All men	Women aged (years):				All women	All
	19–24	25–34	35–49	50–64		19–24	25–34	35–49	50–64		
	cum %	cum %	cum %	cum %	cum %	cum %	cum %	cum %	cum %	cum %	cum %
None	6	1	0	1	1	2	1	1	0	1	1
Less than one portion	38	27	14	7	18	36	19	16	7	16	17
Less than two portions	86	54	36	29	45	64	46	41	20	39	42
Less than three portions	95	76	59	45	64	83	71	61	44	61	62
Less than four portions	95	86	75	60	76	96	82	73	60	74	75
Less than five portions	100	93	86	76	87	96	91	83	78	85	86
All		100	100	100	100	100	100	100	100	100	100
Base	108	219	253	253	833	104	210	318	259	891	1724
Mean number of portions consumed (average value)	1.3	2.2	3.0	3.6	2.7	1.8	2.4	2.9	3.8	2.9	2.8
Median number of portions consumed	1.3	1.8	2.6	3.4	2.2	1.6	2.1	2.4	3.3	2.4	2.3
Standard deviation	1.03	1.61	1.87	2.21	1.99	1.33	1.71	1.98	2.20	2.02	2.01

Note: * Composite dishes were for fruit: fruit pies, and for vegetables: vegetable dishes, including for example vegetable lasagne, cauliflower cheese and vegetable samosas.

Table 2.15(b)

Proportion of respondents consuming portions of fruit, including composite dishes*, by number of portions consumed and sex and age of respondent: fruit (all fruit juice counted as one portion)

Cumulative percentages

Average daily number of portions of fruit consumed	Men aged (years):				All men	Women aged (years):				All women	All
	19–24	25–34	35–49	50–64		19–24	25–34	35–49	50–64		
	cum %	cum %	cum %	cum %	cum %	cum %	cum %	cum %	cum %	cum %	cum %
None	45	27	15	11	21	27	17	17	5	15	18
Less than one portion	79	63	46	38	52	59	54	48	26	44	48
Less than two portions	95	82	71	64	75	86	84	71	56	71	73
Less than three portions	96	91	83	81	86	94	91	85	71	84	85
Less than four portions	100	99	93	89	94	100	97	93	87	93	94
Less than five portions		99	97	94	97		98	98	94	97	97
All		100	100	100	100		100	100	100	100	100
Base	108	219	253	253	833	104	210	318	259	891	1724
Mean number of portions consumed (average value)	0.5	1.0	1.5	1.8	1.3	0.9	1.1	1.4	2.2	1.5	1.4
Median number of portions consumed	0.2	0.6	1.1	1.5	0.9	0.6	0.8	1.0	1.8	1.1	1.0
Standard deviation	0.73	1.13	1.53	1.71	1.48	1.02	1.22	1.42	1.75	1.51	1.50

Note: * Composite dishes were for fruit: fruit pies.

Table 2.15(c)

Proportion of respondents consuming portions of vegetables, including composite dishes*, by number of portions consumed and sex and age of respondent: vegetables (all baked beans and other pulses counted as one portion)

Cumulative percentages

Average daily number of portions of fruit consumed	Men aged (years):				All men	Women aged (years):				All women	All
	19–24	25–34	35–49	50–64		19–24	25–34	35–49	50–64		
	cum %	cum %	cum %	cum %	cum %	cum %	cum %	cum %	cum %	cum %	cum %
None	8	2	0	1	2	3	2	1	1	2	2
Less than one portion	64	48	35	21	38	69	46	38	23	39	38
Less than two portions	98	86	80	62	78	92	83	77	74	80	79
Less than three portions	100	98	92	89	94	100	95	93	94	95	94
Less than four portions		99	99	97	98		99	99	99	99	99
Less than five portions		99	100	99	99		100	100	100	100	100
All		100		100	100						
Base	108	219	253	253	833	104	210	318	259	891	1724
Mean number of portions consumed (average value)	0.8	1.2	1.4	1.8	1.4	0.9	1.2	1.4	1.6	1.4	1.4
Median number of portions consumed	0.7	1.0	1.3	1.6	1.2	0.7	1.1	1.3	1.5	1.2	1.2
Standard deviation	0.60	0.84	0.86	0.98	0.92	0.60	0.88	0.92	0.88	0.89	0.91

Note: * Composite dishes were for vegetables: vegetable dishes, including for example vegetable lasagne, cauliflower cheese and vegetable samosas.

Table 2.16(a)

Proportion of respondents consuming portions of fruit and vegetables, including composite dishes*, by number of portions consumed and region and sex of respondent: fruit and vegetables (all fruit juice counted as one portion; all baked beans and other pulses counted as one portion)

Cumulative percentages

Average daily number of portions of fruit and vegetables consumed	Sex of respondent and region								All
	Men				Women				
	Scotland	Northern	Central, South West and Wales	London and the South East	Scotland	Northern	Central, South West and Wales	London and the South East	
	cum %	cum %	cum %	cum %	cum %	cum %	cum %	cum %	cum %
None	-	2	1	1	1	2	1	0	1
Less than one portion	18	19	20	17	17	25	13	12	17
Less than two portions	44	47	48	40	35	46	40	32	42
Less than three portions	67	67	67	56	60	65	63	54	62
Less than four portions	73	77	78	72	65	76	78	70	75
Less than five portions	83	88	90	83	84	83	87	85	86
All	100	100	100	100	100	100	100	100	100
Base	65	234	294	240	66	229	327	268	1724
Mean number of portions consumed (average value)	2.9	2.6	2.6	3.0	3.0	2.7	2.8	3.2	2.8
Median number of portions consumed	2.4	2.1	2.1	2.6	2.7	2.2	2.3	2.9	2.3
Standard deviation	2.36	1.88	1.88	2.08	1.99	2.13	1.89	2.08	2.01

Note: * Composite dishes were for fruit: fruit pies, and for vegetables: vegetable dishes, including for example vegetable lasagne, cauliflower cheese and vegetable samosas.

Table 2.16(b)

Proportion of respondents consuming portions of fruit, including composite dishes*, by number of portions consumed and region and sex of respondent: fruit (all fruit juice counted as one portion)

Cumulative percentages

Average daily number of portions of fruit consumed	Sex of respondent and region								All
	Men				Women				
	Scotland	Northern	Central, South West and Wales	London and the South East	Scotland	Northern	Central, South West and Wales	London and the South East	
	cum %	cum %	cum %	cum %	cum %	cum %	cum %	cum %	cum %
None	12	22	25	17	10	20	13	13	18
Less than one portion	48	57	57	43	39	50	46	38	48
Less than two portions	73	76	78	71	59	75	75	67	73
Less than three portions	81	85	89	85	73	83	85	85	85
Less than four portions	91	94	94	95	90	91	95	93	94
Less than five portions	94	99	97	97	96	95	98	98	97
All	100	100	100	100	100	100	100	100	100
Base	65	234	294	240	66	229	327	268	1724
Mean number of portions consumed (average value)	1.6	1.2	1.2	1.5	1.8	1.4	1.4	1.6	1.4
Median number of portions consumed	1.1	0.6	0.7	1.1	1.5	1.0	1.1	1.4	1.0
Standard deviation	1.81	1.37	1.44	1.52	1.57	1.65	1.37	1.52	1.50

Note: * Composite dishes were for fruit: fruit pies.

Table 2.16(c)

Proportion of respondents consuming portions of vegetables, including composite dishes*, by number of portions consumed and region and sex of respondent: vegetables (all baked beans and other pulses counted as one portion)

Cumulative percentages

Average daily number of portions of vegetables consumed	Sex of respondent and region								All
	Men				Women				
	Scotland	Northern	Central, South West and Wales	London and the South East	Scotland	Northern	Central, South West and Wales	London and the South East	
	cum %	cum %	cum %	cum %	cum %	cum %	cum %	cum %	cum %
None	-	3	1	2	1	3	2	0	2
Less than one portion	45	37	40	35	51	45	42	28	38
Less than two portions	86	82	77	74	90	81	79	76	79
Less than three portions	94	95	95	91	98	96	95	92	94
Less than four portions	96	99	98	99	100	100	100	98	99
Less than five portions	96	99	100	100				100	100
All	100	100							
Base	65	234	294	240	66	229	327	268	1724
Mean number of portions consumed (average value)	1.3	1.3	1.4	1.5	1.1	1.3	1.3	1.5	1.4
Median number of portions consumed	1.0	1.2	1.2	1.3	1.0	1.1	1.2	1.3	1.2
Standard deviation	1.10	0.89	0.87	0.95	0.74	0.86	0.87	0.95	0.91

Note: * Composite dishes were for vegetables: vegetable dishes, including for example vegetable lasagne, cauliflower cheese and vegetable samosas.

Table 2.17(a)

Proportion of respondents consuming portions of fruit and vegetables, including composite dishes*, by number of portions consumed and whether someone in respondent's household was receiving certain benefits and sex of respondent: fruit and vegetables (all fruit juice counted as one portion; all baked beans and other pulses counted as one portion)

Cumulative percentages

Average daily number of portions of fruit and vegetables consumed	Sex of respondent and whether receiving benefits								All
	Men				**Women**				
	Scotland	Northern	Central, South West and Wales	London and the South East	Scotland	Northern	Central, South West and Wales	London and the South East	
		cum %		cum %		cum %		cum %	cum %
None		3		1		4		0	1
Less than one portion		27		17		36		12	17
Less than two portions		65		42		67		33	42
Less than three portions		81		61		83		56	62
Less than four portions		88		74		88		71	75
Less than five portions		91		86		96		83	86
All		100		100		100		100	100
Base		*110*		*723*		*150*		*741*	*1724*
Mean number of portions consumed (average value)		2.1		2.8		1.9		3.1	2.8
Median number of portions consumed		1.6		2.4		1.4		2.8	2.3
Standard deviation		1.97		1.97		1.72		2.02	2.01

Note: ** Composite dishes were for fruit: fruit pies, and for vegetables: vegetable dishes, including for example vegetable lasagne, cauliflower cheese and vegetable samosas.*

Table 2.17(b)

Proportion of respondents consuming portions of fruit, including composite dishes*, by number of portions consumed and whether someone in respondent's household was receiving certain benefits and sex of respondent: fruit (all fruit juice counted as one portion)

Cumulative percentages

Average daily number of portions of fruit consumed	Sex of respondent and whether receiving benefits								All
	Men				**Women**				
	Scotland	Northern	Central, South West and Wales	London and the South East	Scotland	Northern	Central, South West and Wales	London and the South East	
		cum %		cum %		cum %		cum %	cum %
None		35		19		30		12	18
Less than one portion		70		49		66		40	48
Less than two portions		86		73		86		68	73
Less than three portions		92		85		92		82	85
Less than four portions		95		94		97		92	94
Less than five portions		96		97		98		97	97
All		100		100		100		100	100
Base		*110*		*723*		*150*		*741*	*1724*
Mean number of portions consumed (average value)		0.9		1.4		0.9		1.6	1.4
Median number of portions consumed		0.4		1.0		0.5		1.2	1.0
Standard deviation		1.34		1.49		1.40		1.50	1.50

Note: ** Composite dishes were for fruit: fruit pies.*

Table 2.17(c)

Proportion of respondents consuming portions of vegetables, including composite dishes*, by number of portions consumed and whether someone in respondent's household was receiving certain benefits and sex of respondent: vegetables (all baked beans and other pulses counted as one portion)

Cumulative percentages

Average daily number of portions of vegetables consumed	Sex of respondent and whether receiving benefits								All
	Men				Women				
	Scotland	Northern	Central, South West and Wales	London and the South East	Scotland	Northern	Central, South West and Wales	London and the South East	
		cum %		cum %		cum %		cum %	cum %
None		4		2		6		1	2
Less than one portion		49		36		59		35	38
Less than two portions		87		77		94		76	79
Less than three portions		93		94		100		94	94
Less than four portions		100		98				99	99
Less than five portions				99				100	100
All				100					
Base		110		723		150		741	1724
Mean number of portions consumed (average value)		1.2		1.4		0.9		1.4	1.4
Median number of portions consumed		1.0		1.2		0.9		1.3	1.2
Standard deviation		0.85		0.93		0.70		0.90	0.91

Note: * Composite dishes were for vegetables: vegetable dishes, including for example vegetable lasagne, cauliflower cheese and vegetable samosas.

Appendix A   Fruit and vegetables

1   Definitions

Fruit and vegetable intake was defined in a number of different ways. In total 18 variables were derived. For each variable, the average daily intake in grams and the average daily number of portions consumed were calculated. The following sections explain the derivation of these variables and Table A1 provides a summary of each variable.

1.1   Fruit and fruit juice

Fruit comprised food groups apples & pears, citrus fruits, bananas, canned fruit in juice, canned fruit in syrup, and 'other fruit' (for example plums, grapes and soft fruits), together with fruit juice. Fruit juice includes vegetable juices. Quantities consumed in each of these food groups over the seven-day dietary recording period were added and then divided by seven to give an average daily intake of fruit in grams. This was then divided by 80 to give an average daily number of portions consumed.

Fruit juice was not included in the first variable calculated for fruit. In the second variable, only one portion of fruit juice a day was included, however much was consumed. Thus, if the respondent consumed a daily average of at least 80g of fruit juice this counted as one portion and a value of 80g was added to the average daily amount of fruit consumed. The third definition includes all fruit juice, irrespective of the amount consumed.

These three variables were calculated excluding and then including composite dishes, in this instance, fruit pies. As fruit is not the only component of fruit pies, the fruit contribution from fruit pies was estimated as 45% of the total weight, including the pastry. Fruit contained in other products such as yogurts, jams, fruit smoothies, sponge puddings, cakes, breakfast cereals and crumbles was not included in the derivation of fruit intake.

1.2   Vegetables and pulses

Vegetables comprised food groups raw carrots, raw tomatoes, 'other raw' & salad vegetables, peas, green beans, leafy green vegetables, carrots – not raw, tomatoes – not raw, 'other vegetables' and baked beans. In line with the definitions used in the five-a-day programme, potatoes and similar starchy staples (such as plantain and yam) do not count towards vegetable intake and are excluded from these derivations. The 'other vegetables' food group includes vegetables such as mushrooms, cauliflower, onions and peppers, as well as starchy staple vegetables and soya-based food items that are used as meat alternatives. As these soya-based foods and starchy staple vegetables do not count towards intake of vegetables in this context, these items[1] were excluded at food code level. The food groups peas and 'other vegetables' include pulses, and these are not included in all the derivations of vegetable intake. New groups were therefore derived which excluded pulses, and which comprised pulses only.

Quantities consumed in each of these food groups over the seven-day dietary recording period were added together and then divided by seven to give an average daily intake of vegetables in grams. This was then divided by 80 to give an average daily number of portions consumed.

Baked beans and other pulses were not included in the first variable calculated for vegetables. In the second variable, one portion only of baked beans and other pulses was included. Thus, if the respondent consumed a daily average of at least 80g of baked beans and other pulses this would count as one portion and a value of 80g added to the average daily amount of vegetables consumed. The third definition includes all baked beans and other pulses consumed, irrespective of the amount.

These three variables were calculated excluding composite dishes, and then including composite dishes, in this instance, vegetable dishes. As vegetables are not the only component in vegetable dishes (for example potatoes in vegetable curry) the vegetable contribution from vegetable dishes was estimated as 40% of the consumed weight. Vegetables contained in other products such as soups, quiches, omelettes, pizzas and meat dishes (for example stews and casseroles) and tomato ketchup were not included in the derivation of vegetable intake.

1.3   Fruit and vegetables

The same definitions were used in the calculations of combined fruit and vegetable intake. The first derivation of fruit and vegetables excludes fruit juice and baked beans and other pulses; the second includes one portion only of fruit juice and baked beans and other pulses; and the third definition includes all fruit juice and baked beans and other pulses.

2   Quantities of fruit and vegetables consumed

Tables A2(a) to A7(b) show the proportion of respondents consuming fruit and vegetables during the seven-day dietary recording period, together with the mean and median amounts consumed daily by all respondents including non-consumers, and by consumers only. Data are presented for men and women by age group, by region and by receipt of benefits. Table A8 shows mean and median amounts consumed for all consumers and all respondents, for men and women combined.

These tables show consumption of fruit and vegetables for each of the 18 different variables (as discussed earlier on pages 16–19, and shown in Table A1). They, therefore, allow the reader to see the proportions of respondents who ate fruit, the proportions who ate vegetables, and the differences that the inclusion of composite dishes

and all portions of fruit juice, baked beans and other pulses make to the amounts of fruit and vegetables consumed daily.

References and endnotes

1   The excluded food items from the 'other vegetables' category were:

> green bananas
> yam
> plantain
> soya mince
> soya bean curd tofu
> bacon flavoured TVP strips
> Cheatin' meats (eg ham, chicken)
> Quorn

Table A1

Summary of fruit, vegetable, and fruit and vegetable variables

Variable	Included foods	Excluded foods
Fruit		
(1) Fruit	Apples and pears Citrus fruits Bananas Canned fruit in juice Canned fruit in syrup Other fruit e.g. grapes and plums	Fruit juice Composite dishes (fruit pies)
(2) Fruit including 1 portion fruit juice	As (1) above One portion of fruit juice (80g)	Fruit juice if less than average of 80g consumed daily Fruit juice in excess of 80g consumed daily Composite dishes (fruit pies)
(3) Fruit including all fruit juice	As (1) above All fruit juice	Composite dishes (fruit pies)
(4) Fruit including composite dishes	As (1) above Fruit pies, 45% total weight	Fruit juice

(5) Fruit including composite dishes and
    1 portion fruit juice
	As (2) above
	Fruit pies, 45% total weight
		Fruit juice if less than average of 80g
		    consumed daily
		Fruit juice in excess of 80g consumed daily

(6) Fruit including composite dishes and all fruit juice	As (3) above Fruit pies, 45% total weight	
Vegetables		

(7) Vegetables	Raw carrots
	Raw tomatoes
	Other raw and salad vegetables
	Peas
	Green beans
	Leafy green vegetables
	Carrots – not raw
	Tomatoes – not raw
	Other vegetables
		From other vegetables*:
		    Green bananas
		    Yam
		    Plantain
		    Soya mince
		    Soya bean curd tofu
		    Bacon flavoured TVP strips
		    Cheatin' meats (eg ham)
		    Quorn
		Baked beans
		Pulses (from peas and other vegetables)

(8) Vegetables including 1 portion baked beans
    and other pulses
	As (7) above
	One portion of baked beans and other pulses
		Baked beans and other pulses if less than
		    average of 80g consumed daily
		Baked beans and other pulses in excess of
		    80g consumed daily
		Composite dishes (vegetable dishes)

(9) Vegetables including all baked beans and other pulses	As (7) above All baked beans and other pulses	Composite dishes (vegetable dishes)
(10) Vegetables including composite dishes	As (7) above Vegetable dishes, 40% total weight	Baked beans Pulses

(11) Vegetables including composite dishes
    and 1 portion baked beans and other pulses
	As (8) above
	Vegetable dishes, 40% total weight
		Baked beans and other pulses if less than
		    average of 80g consumed daily
		Baked beans and other pulses in excess of
		    80g consumed daily

(12) Vegetables including composite dishes and all baked beans and other pulses	As (9) above Vegetable dishes, 40% total weight	
Fruit and vegetables		
(13) Fruit and vegetables	(1) and (7) above combined	As for (1) and (7) above
(14) Fruit and vegetables including 1 portion fruit juice and/or baked beans and other pulses	(2) and (8) above combined	As for (2) and (8) above
(15) Fruit and vegetables including all fruit juice and baked beans and other pulses	(3) and (9) above combined	As for (3) and (9) above
(16) Fruit and vegetables including composite dishes	(4) and (10) above combined	As for (4) and (10) above

(17) Fruit and vegetables including composite
    dishes and 1 portion fruit juice and/or
    baked beans and other pulses
	(5) and (11) above combined	As for (5) and (11) above

(18) Fruit and vegetables including composite
    dishes and all fruit juice and baked beans
    and other pulses
	(6) and (12) above combined	As for (6) and (12) above

Note: * These items were excluded from all derivations of vegetable intake.

Table A2(a)

Average daily amount (grams) of fruit and vegetables consumed by age of respondent: men, including non-consumers

Grams

Fruit and vegetables	All men aged (years):								All men	
	19–24		25–34		35–49		50–64			
	Mean	sd	Mean	sd	Mean	sd	Mean	sd	Mean	sd
	g	g	g	g	g	g	g	g	g	g
Excluding composite dishes:										
Fruit, no fruit juice	27	42	61	76	99	110	122	123	87	105
Fruit including one portion fruit juice	38	58	76	89	119	122	143	137	105	118
Fruit including all fruit juice	65	110	98	113	156	165	177	170	135	153
Vegetables, no baked beans/pulses	53	42	85	65	102	62	136	76	102	71
Vegetables including one portion baked beans and other pulses	62	47	88	65	108	66	138	77	106	72
Vegetables including all baked beans and other pulses	88	69	105	68	125	70	151	78	123	75
Fruit and vegetables, no fruit juice or baked beans/pulses	80	70	146	113	202	133	258	162	188	144
Fruit and vegetables (including one portion fruit juice, and/or one portion baked beans and other pulses)	102	83	164	125	228	146	282	174	211	156
Fruit and vegetables (including all fruit juice and all baked beans and other pulses)	153	133	203	151	281	185	328	205	258	188
Including composite dishes*:										
Fruit, no fruit juice	28	42	62	77	100	110	124	123	88	106
Fruit including one portion fruit juice	38	58	78	90	120	122	146	137	106	119
Fruit including all fruit juice	65	110	99	114	157	165	180	170	137	154
Vegetables, no baked beans/pulses	56	42	92	67	109	65	140	78	107	72
Vegetables including one portion baked beans and other pulses	65	48	94	67	115	69	142	78	111	74
Vegetables including all baked beans and other pulses	91	70	111	69	132	72	155	79	128	76
Fruit and vegetables, no fruit juice or baked beans/pulses	84	70	154	116	210	136	264	165	195	147
Fruit and vegetables (including one portion fruit juice, and/or one portion baked beans and other pulses)	105	82	172	128	236	150	288	177	218	159
Fruit and vegetables (including all fruit juice and all baked beans and other pulses)	156	134	211	155	289	189	335	208	265	191
Base = number of respondents		108		219		253		253		833

Note: * Composite dishes were for fruit: fruit pies, and for vegetables: vegetable dishes, including for example vegetable lasagne, cauliflower cheese and vegetable samosas.

Table A2(b)

Average daily amount (grams) of fruit and vegetables consumed by age of respondent: women, including non-consumers

Grams

Fruit and vegetables	All women aged (years):								All women	
	19–24		25–34		35–49		50–64			
	Mean	sd	Mean	sd	Mean	sd	Mean	sd	Mean	sd
	g	g	g	g	g	g	g	g	g	g
Excluding composite dishes:										
Fruit, no fruit juice	54	67	74	88	98	105	151	136	103	113
Fruit including one portion fruit juice	73	81	90	97	114	114	171	140	120	120
Fruit including all fruit juice	104	110	120	120	141	141	203	167	150	146
Vegetables, no baked beans/pulses	62	46	87	68	104	69	120	67	100	68
Vegetables including one portion baked beans and other pulses	63	46	89	68	105	70	121	68	101	69
Vegetables including all baked beans and other pulses	75	52	103	69	117	72	130	68	113	70
Fruit and vegetables, no fruit juice or baked beans/pulses	116	94	162	127	202	147	272	170	203	153
Fruit and vegetables (including one portion fruit juice, and/or one portion baked beans and other pulses)	136	106	182	135	220	155	294	173	222	160
Fruit and vegetables (including all fruit juice and all baked beans and other pulses)	179	134	223	153	258	178	333	198	262	181
Including composite dishes*:										
Fruit, no fruit juice	54	67	75	88	99	104	153	136	104	113
Fruit including one portion fruit juice	73	81	91	97	115	114	172	140	121	121
Fruit including all fruit juice	105	110	120	120	142	141	204	168	151	146
Vegetables, no baked beans/pulses	67	47	98	70	112	72	125	70	107	71
Vegetables including one portion baked beans and other pulses	68	48	99	71	114	73	126	71	109	71
Vegetables including all baked beans and other pulses	81	52	114	73	125	75	135	71	120	73
Fruit and vegetables, no fruit juice or baked beans/pulses	122	94	173	129	211	149	278	173	211	155
Fruit and vegetables (including one portion fruit juice, and/or one portion baked beans and other pulses)	142	106	193	137	229	158	300	176	231	162
Fruit and vegetables (including all fruit juice and all baked beans and other pulses)	185	133	234	155	267	181	340	201	271	184
Base = number of respondents		104		210		318		259		891

Note: * Composite dishes were for fruit: fruit pies, and for vegetables: vegetable dishes, including for example vegetable lasagne, cauliflower cheese and vegetable samosas.

Table A3(a)

Average daily amount (grams) of fruit and vegetables consumed by age of respondent: men consumers

Fruit and vegetables	Men consumers aged (years):								
	19–24			25–34			35–49		
	Mean	Median	% consumers	Mean	Median	% consumers	Mean	Median	% consumers
	g	g		g	g		g	g	
Excluding composite dishes:									
Fruit, no fruit juice	58	48	46	90	68	68	119	92	83
Fruit including one portion fruit juice	72	57	53	108	80	71	141	108	84
Fruit including all fruit juice	110	74	59	124	86	79	181	133	86
Vegetables, no baked beans/pulses	58	47	93	87	76	98	103	93	100
Vegetables including one portion baked beans and other pulses	67	60	93	90	78	98	109	96	100
Vegetables including all baked beans and other pulses	91	82	96	106	98	99	125	111	100
Fruit and vegetables, no fruit juice or baked beans/pulses	87	65	93	149	130	99	202	178	100
Fruit and vegetables (including one portion fruit juice, and/or one portion baked beans and other pulses)	108	111	94	166	142	99	229	201	100
Fruit and vegetables (including all fruit juice and all baked beans and other pulses)	158	127	96	204	165	100	281	247	100
Including composite dishes*:									
Fruit, no fruit juice	57	48	49	87	63	72	120	91	84
Fruit including one portion fruit juice	70	56	56	106	80	74	141	110	85
Fruit including all fruit juice	107	59	61	125	85	79	181	134	87
Vegetables, no baked beans/pulses	61	53	93	94	83	98	109	97	100
Vegetables including one portion baked beans and other pulses	70	67	93	96	86	98	115	102	100
Vegetables including all baked beans and other pulses	94	87	96	113	101	99	132	118	100
Fruit and vegetables, no fruit juice or baked beans/pulses	90	68	93	156	134	99	210	186	100
Fruit and vegetables (including one portion fruit juice, and/or one portion baked beans and other pulses)	112	111	94	174	150	99	237	210	100
Fruit and vegetables (including all fruit juice and all baked beans and other pulses)	162	138	96	212	173	100	289	247	100
Base = number of respondents			108			219			253

Note: * Composite dishes were for fruit: fruit pies, and for vegetables: vegetable dishes, including for example vegetable lasagne, cauliflower cheese and vegetable samosas.

Grams and percentages

50–64			All men			
Mean	Median	% consumers	Mean	Median	% consumers	
g	g		g	g		
						Excluding composite dishes:
141	120	87	115	84	75	Fruit, no fruit juice
163	137	88	134	99	78	Fruit including one portion fruit juice
201	155	88	166	122	81	Fruit including all fruit juice
137	124	99	104	90	98	Vegetables, no baked beans/pulses
139	125	99	108	94	98	Vegetables including one portion baked beans and other pulses
152	140	100	124	113	99	Vegetables including all baked beans and other pulses
260	234	99	192	155	98	Fruit and vegetables, no fruit juice or baked beans/pulses
283	264	100	214	175	99	Fruit and vegetables (including one portion fruit juice, and/or one portion baked beans and other pulses)
329	295	100	260	215	99	Fruit and vegetables (including all fruit juice and all baked beans and other pulses)
						Including composite dishes*:
142	120	88	114	83	77	Fruit, no fruit juice
164	137	88	134	100	79	Fruit including one portion fruit juice
202	158	89	166	124	82	Fruit including all fruit juice
142	128	99	109	94	98	Vegetables, no baked beans/pulses
143	128	99	113	98	98	Vegetables including one portion baked beans and other pulses
156	144	100	130	119	99	Vegetables including all baked beans and other pulses
266	237	99	198	162	98	Fruit and vegetables, no fruit juice or baked beans/pulses
290	271	100	221	180	99	Fruit and vegetables (including one portion fruit juice, and/or one portion baked beans and other pulses)
336	305	100	267	219	99	Fruit and vegetables (including all fruit juice and all baked beans and other pulses)
		253			833	*Base = number of respondents*

Table A3(b)

Average daily amount (grams) of fruit and vegetables consumed by age of respondent: women consumers

Fruit and vegetables	Women consumers aged (years):								
	19–24			25–34			35–49		
	Mean	Median	% consumers	Mean	Median	% consumers	Mean	Median	% consumers
	g	g		g	g		g	g	
Excluding composite dishes:									
Fruit, no fruit juice	79	58	69	93	63	80	122	93	80
Fruit including one portion fruit juice	101	82	73	110	84	82	139	112	82
Fruit including all fruit juice	131	98	80	137	97	87	167	141	84
Vegetables, no baked beans/pulses	66	51	94	90	72	97	106	95	98
Vegetables including one portion baked beans and other pulses	67	53	94	92	78	97	107	95	98
Vegetables including all baked beans and other pulses	78	63	96	105	90	99	119	108	98
Fruit and vegetables, no fruit juice or baked beans/pulses	121	99	96	164	129	99	204	170	99
Fruit and vegetables (including one portion fruit juice, and/or one portion baked beans and other pulses)	140	109	97	185	163	99	222	185	99
Fruit and vegetables (including all fruit juice and all baked beans and other pulses)	181	135	99	225	191	100	260	218	99
Including composite dishes*:									
Fruit, no fruit juice	78	57	70	92	65	81	122	91	81
Fruit including one portion fruit juice	101	86	73	110	84	83	138	111	83
Fruit including all fruit juice	132	98	80	138	97	88	167	140	85
Vegetables, no baked beans/pulses	70	58	97	100	86	98	114	105	99
Vegetables including one portion baked beans and other pulses	71	64	97	102	88	98	115	106	99
Vegetables including all baked beans and other pulses	82	70	98	115	103	99	126	115	99
Fruit and vegetables, no fruit juice or baked beans/pulses	126	105	97	175	144	99	213	175	99
Fruit and vegetables (including one portion fruit juice, and/or one portion baked beans and other pulses)	145	126	98	195	169	99	231	195	99
Fruit and vegetables (including all fruit juice and all baked beans and other pulses)	187	166	99	234	202	100	269	227	99
Base = number of respondents			104			210			318

Note: * Composite dishes were for fruit: fruit pies, and for vegetables: vegetable dishes, including for example vegetable lasagne, cauliflower cheese and vegetable samosas.

NDNS adults aged 19 to 64, Volume 1 2002

Grams and percentages

50–64			All women			
Mean	Median	% consumers	Mean	Median	% consumers	
g	g		g	g		**Excluding composite dishes:**
163	136	93	124	90	83	Fruit, no fruit juice
181	145	94	142	114	85	Fruit including one portion fruit juice
213	173	95	171	133	88	Fruit including all fruit juice
121	112	99	102	91	98	Vegetables, no baked beans/pulses
122	112	99	103	93	98	Vegetables including one portion baked beans and other pulses
131	129	100	114	105	98	Vegetables including all baked beans and other pulses
272	237	100	205	170	99	Fruit and vegetables, no fruit juice or baked beans/pulses
294	263	100	225	187	99	Fruit and vegetables (including one portion fruit juice, and/or one portion baked beans and other pulses)
334	299	100	264	223	99	Fruit and vegetables (including all fruit juice and all baked beans and other pulses)
						Including composite dishes*:
164	135	93	124	90	84	Fruit, no fruit juice
182	152	95	142	113	85	Fruit including one portion fruit juice
214	180	95	171	133	88	Fruit including all fruit juice
126	121	99	109	98	98	Vegetables, no baked beans/pulses
127	121	99	110	99	98	Vegetables including one portion baked beans and other pulses
136	133	100	121	110	99	Vegetables including all baked beans and other pulses
279	244	100	213	173	99	Fruit and vegetables, no fruit juice or baked beans/pulses
301	265	100	233	196	99	Fruit and vegetables (including one portion fruit juice, and/or one portion baked beans and other pulses)
340	306	100	272	230	100	Fruit and vegetables (including all fruit juice and all baked beans and other pulses)
		259			891	*Base = number of respondents*

Table A4(a)

Average daily amount (grams) of fruit and vegetables consumed by region: men, including non-consumers

Grams

Fruit and vegetables	Region							
	Scotland		Northern		Central, South West and Wales		London and the South East	
	Mean	sd	Mean	sd	Mean	sd	Mean	sd
	g	g	g	g	g	g	g	g
Excluding composite dishes:								
Fruit, no fruit juice	109	129	79	97	80	101	97	109
Fruit including one portion fruit juice	126	143	96	110	95	115	118	121
Fruit including all fruit juice	156	172	120	146	120	143	162	164
Vegetables, no baked beans/pulses	102	89	98	69	100	66	107	73
Vegetables including one portion baked beans and other pulses	103	89	102	71	106	68	110	74
Vegetables including all baked beans and other pulses	116	87	120	74	124	73	126	76
Fruit and vegetables, no fruit juice or baked beans/pulses	211	176	177	134	180	138	204	151
Fruit and vegetables (including one portion fruit juice, and/or one portion baked beans and other pulses)	229	188	201	149	202	148	229	162
Fruit and vegetables (including all fruit juice and all baked beans and other pulses)	272	215	240	186	245	175	288	195
Including composite dishes*:								
Fruit, no fruit juice	111	131	80	97	81	102	98	109
Fruit including one portion fruit juice	127	145	97	110	97	115	120	122
Fruit including all fruit juice	157	174	122	146	122	143	164	164
Vegetables, no baked beans/pulses	105	88	102	69	104	68	116	75
Vegetables including one portion baked beans and other pulses	106	88	106	71	110	70	119	76
Vegetables including all baked beans and other pulses	119	86	124	74	128	74	135	79
Fruit and vegetables, no fruit juice or baked beans/pulses	216	176	182	136	185	141	215	154
Fruit and vegetables (including one portion fruit juice, and/or one portion baked beans and other pulses)	234	189	206	151	207	151	240	166
Fruit and vegetables (including all fruit juice and all baked beans and other pulses)	276	216	246	186	250	178	299	199
Base = number of respondents		65		234		294		240

Note: * Composite dishes were for fruit: fruit pies, and for vegetables: vegetable dishes, including for example vegetable lasagne, cauliflower cheese and vegetable samosas.

Table A4(b)

Average daily amount (grams) of fruit and vegetables consumed by region: women, including non-consumers

Grams

Fruit and vegetables	Region							
	Scotland		Northern		Central, South West and Wales		London and the South East	
	Mean	sd	Mean	sd	Mean	sd	Mean	sd
	g	g	g	g	g	g	g	g
Excluding composite dishes:								
Fruit, no fruit juice	121	110	98	124	97	99	110	118
Fruit including one portion fruit juice	145	126	113	132	114	110	128	121
Fruit including all fruit juice	191	178	136	147	142	137	160	144
Vegetables, no baked beans/pulses	84	60	96	66	99	66	108	72
Vegetables including one portion baked beans and other pulses	85	60	97	67	101	67	109	74
Vegetables including all baked beans and other pulses	94	60	110	68	113	69	120	75
Fruit and vegetables, no fruit juice or baked beans/pulses	205	142	194	161	196	142	218	162
Fruit and vegetables (including one portion fruit juice, and/or one portion baked beans and other pulses)	232	158	212	169	215	149	238	165
Fruit and vegetables (including all fruit juice and all baked beans and other pulses)	285	206	245	182	255	172	280	184
Including composite dishes*:								
Fruit, no fruit juice	121	110	99	124	98	100	111	118
Fruit including one portion fruit juice	145	126	114	132	114	110	129	121
Fruit including all fruit juice	192	178	137	148	143	137	161	144
Vegetables, no baked beans/pulses	88	59	100	68	105	69	121	75
Vegetables including one portion baked beans and other pulses	89	59	101	69	107	70	122	76
Vegetables including all baked beans and other pulses	98	59	114	70	119	72	132	78
Fruit and vegetables, no fruit juice or baked beans/pulses	210	143	199	163	203	144	231	164
Fruit and vegetables (including one portion fruit juice, and/or one portion baked beans and other pulses)	236	159	218	170	222	152	252	166
Fruit and vegetables (including all fruit juice and all baked beans and other pulses)	289	206	251	184	262	175	293	186
Base = number of respondents		66		229		327		268

Note: * Composite dishes were for fruit: fruit pies, and for vegetables: vegetable dishes, including for example vegetable lasagne, cauliflower cheese and vegetable samosas.

Table A5(a)

Average daily amount (grams) of fruit and vegetables consumed by region: men consumers

Grams and percentages

Fruit and vegetables	Region											
	Scotland			Northern			Central, South West and Wales			London and the South East		
	Mean	Median	% consumers	Mean	Median	% consumers	Mean	Median	% consumers	Mean	Median	% consumers
	g	g		g	g		g	g		g	g	
Excluding composite dishes:												
Fruit, no fruit juice	128	97	86	109	73	73	110	78	72	122	93	79
Fruit including one portion fruit juice	148	111	86	128	92	75	129	89	74	143	111	82
Fruit including all fruit juice	181	133	86	152	98	79	154	115	78	189	142	86
Vegetables, no baked beans/pulses	102	81	100	101	92	97	102	88	98	109	94	98
Vegetables including one portion baked beans and other pulses	103	81	100	105	95	97	108	94	99	112	99	98
Vegetables including all baked beans and other pulses	116	94	100	121	114	100	126	114	99	128	118	99
Fruit and vegetables, no fruit juice or baked beans/pulses	211	158	100	181	143	98	183	146	98	206	179	99
Fruit and vegetables (including one portion fruit juice, and/or one portion baked beans and other pulses)	229	188	100	204	161	98	204	170	99	232	205	99
Fruit and vegetables (including all fruit juice and all baked beans and other pulses)	272	218	100	242	190	100	247	211	99	291	254	99
Including composite dishes*:												
Fruit, no fruit juice	126	90	88	106	73	76	109	76	74	123	91	80
Fruit including one portion fruit juice	146	110	88	125	90	78	129	92	75	144	117	83
Fruit including all fruit juice	178	132	89	151	97	81	154	113	79	191	143	86
Vegetables, no baked beans/pulses	105	83	100	105	96	97	106	90	98	119	103	98
Vegetables including one portion baked beans and other pulses	106	83	100	110	97	97	111	100	99	122	108	98
Vegetables including all baked beans and other pulses	119	97	100	125	120	100	129	119	99	137	124	99
Fruit and vegetables, no fruit juice or baked beans/pulses	216	166	100	187	156	98	188	150	98	218	192	99
Fruit and vegetables (including one portion fruit juice, and/or one portion baked beans and other pulses)	234	192	100	210	169	98	209	172	99	243	211	99
Fruit and vegetables (including all fruit juice and all baked beans and other pulses)	276	218	100	247	197	100	252	213	99	302	267	99
Base = number of respondents			65			234			294			240

Note: * Composite dishes were for fruit: fruit pies, and for vegetables: vegetable dishes, including for example vegetable lasagne, cauliflower cheese and vegetable samosas.

Table A5(b)

Average daily amount (grams) of fruit and vegetables consumed by region: women consumers

Grams and percentages

Fruit and vegetables	Region											
	Scotland			Northern			Central, South West and Wales			London and the South East		
	Mean	Median	% consumers	Mean	Median	% consumers	Mean	Median	% consumers	Mean	Median	% consumers
	g	g		g	g		g	g		g	g	
Excluding composite dishes:												
Fruit, no fruit juice	135	93	89	126	88	78	114	82	85	132	109	83
Fruit including one portion fruit juice	162	139	89	144	99	79	131	103	86	149	129	86
Fruit including all fruit juice	208	158	91	164	117	83	160	117	89	180	154	89
Vegetables, no baked beans/pulses	86	78	97	99	90	97	101	88	98	110	101	98
Vegetables including one portion baked beans and other pulses	87	79	97	100	90	97	102	90	98	112	101	98
Vegetables including all baked beans and other pulses	95	92	98	111	100	99	115	105	98	122	112	98
Fruit and vegetables, no fruit juice or baked beans/pulses	210	175	97	198	155	98	198	166	99	219	188	100
Fruit and vegetables (including one portion fruit juice, and/or one portion baked beans and other pulses)	237	212	97	216	171	98	217	176	99	240	216	100
Fruit and vegetables (including all fruit juice and all baked beans and other pulses)	288	224	98	247	197	100	257	215	99	282	259	100
Including composite dishes*:												
Fruit, no fruit juice	134	93	89	126	86	79	115	83	85	131	108	84
Fruit including one portion fruit juice	161	139	89	144	100	80	132	102	87	148	129	87
Fruit including all fruit juice	207	157	92	164	116	83	160	116	90	181	154	89
Vegetables, no baked beans/pulses	89	79	98	103	91	97	107	95	98	121	107	100
Vegetables including one portion baked beans and other pulses	90	81	98	104	92	97	109	98	98	122	107	100
Vegetables including all baked beans and other pulses	99	95	98	115	102	100	121	109	98	133	118	100
Fruit and vegetables, no fruit juice or baked beans/pulses	212	170	98	202	159	99	206	170	99	232	196	100
Fruit and vegetables (including one portion fruit juice, and/or one portion baked beans and other pulses)	239	214	98	221	175	99	224	183	99	252	232	100
Fruit and vegetables (including all fruit juice and all baked beans and other pulses)	292	225	98	251	203	100	264	225	99	294	270	100
Base = number of respondents		66			229			327			268	

Note: * Composite dishes were for fruit: fruit pies, and for vegetables: vegetable dishes, including for example vegetable lasagne, cauliflower cheese and vegetable samosas.

Table A6(a)

Average daily amount (grams) of fruit and vegetables consumed by whether someone in respondent's household was receiving certain benefits: men, including non-consumers

Grams

Fruit and vegetables	Whether receiving benefits			
	Receiving benefits		Not receiving benefits	
	Mean	sd	Mean	sd
	g	g	g	g
Excluding composite dishes:				
Fruit, no fruit juice	57	95	91	106
Fruit including one portion fruit juice	70	107	110	119
Fruit including all fruit juice	84	126	143	156
Vegetables, no baked beans/pulses	87	65	104	71
Vegetables including one portion baked beans and other pulses	91	66	108	73
Vegetables including all baked beans and other pulses	109	71	125	76
Fruit and vegetables, no fruit juice or baked beans/pulses	145	143	195	143
Fruit and vegetables (including one portion fruit juice, and/or one portion baked beans and other pulses)	163	155	219	155
Fruit and vegetables (including all fruit juice and all baked beans and other pulses)	194	171	268	188
Including composite dishes*:				
Fruit, no fruit juice	58	96	93	106
Fruit including one portion fruit juice	71	108	111	120
Fruit including all fruit juice	85	127	145	156
Vegetables, no baked beans/pulses	91	67	109	73
Vegetables including one portion baked beans and other pulses	95	68	114	74
Vegetables including all baked beans and other pulses	113	72	130	77
Fruit and vegetables, no fruit juice or baked beans/pulses	150	144	202	146
Fruit and vegetables (including one portion fruit juice, and/or one portion baked beans and other pulses)	168	158	226	158
Fruit and vegetables (including all fruit juice and all baked beans and other pulses)	199	173	275	192
Base = number of respondents		110		723

Note: * Composite dishes were for fruit: fruit pies, and for vegetables: vegetable dishes, including for example vegetable lasagne, cauliflower cheese and vegetable samosas.

Table A6(b)

Average daily amount (grams) of fruit and vegetables consumed by whether someone in respondent's household was receiving certain benefits: women, including non-consumers

Grams

Fruit and vegetables	Whether receiving benefits			
	Receiving benefits		Not receiving benefits	
	Mean	sd	Mean	sd
	g	g	g	g
Excluding composite dishes:				
Fruit, no fruit juice	60	104	112	113
Fruit including one portion fruit juice	74	112	129	120
Fruit including all fruit juice	108	156	158	142
Vegetables, no baked beans/pulses	67	53	106	69
Vegetables including one portion baked beans and other pulses	69	55	108	70
Vegetables including all baked beans and other pulses	81	57	119	71
Fruit and vegetables, no fruit juice or baked beans/pulses	128	128	218	154
Fruit and vegetables (including one portion fruit juice, and/or one portion baked beans and other pulses)	144	136	238	160
Fruit and vegetables (including all fruit juice and all baked beans and other pulses)	188	177	277	179
Including composite dishes*:				
Fruit, no fruit juice	61	104	112	113
Fruit including one portion fruit juice	75	112	130	120
Fruit including all fruit juice	108	156	159	142
Vegetables, no baked beans/pulses	73	54	114	72
Vegetables including one portion baked beans and other pulses	75	56	115	72
Vegetables including all baked beans and other pulses	86	58	127	74
Fruit and vegetables, no fruit juice or baked beans/pulses	134	129	227	156
Fruit and vegetables (including one portion fruit juice, and/or one portion baked beans and other pulses)	150	137	247	162
Fruit and vegetables (including all fruit juice and all baked beans and other pulses)	195	179	286	181
Base = number of respondents		150		741

Note: *Composite dishes were for fruit: fruit pies, and for vegetables: vegetable dishes, including for example vegetable lasagne, cauliflower cheese and vegetable samosas.*

Table A7(a)

Average daily amount (grams) of fruit and vegetables consumed by whether someone in respondent's household was receiving certain benefits: men consumers

Grams and percentages

Fruit and vegetables	Whether receiving benefits					
	Receiving benefits			Not receiving benefits		
	Mean	Median	% consumers	Mean	Median	% consumers
	g	g		g	g	
Excluding composite dishes:						
Fruit, no fruit juice	97	58	59	117	87	78
Fruit including one portion fruit juice	110	73	64	138	106	80
Fruit including all fruit juice	124	69	68	172	130	83
Vegetables, no baked beans/pulses	92	79	94	106	91	98
Vegetables including one portion baked beans and other pulses	95	85	96	110	96	98
Vegetables including all baked beans and other pulses	110	102	99	126	115	99
Fruit and vegetables, no fruit juice or baked beans/pulses	152	112	95	197	165	99
Fruit and vegetables (including one portion fruit juice, and/or one portion baked beans and other pulses)	169	133	96	221	186	99
Fruit and vegetables (including all fruit juice and all baked beans and other pulses)	195	152	99	270	230	99
Including composite dishes*:						
Fruit, no fruit juice	94	54	62	116	87	80
Fruit including one portion fruit juice	110	75	64	137	108	81
Fruit including all fruit juice	124	74	68	172	130	84
Vegetables, no baked beans/pulses	96	84	94	111	97	98
Vegetables including one portion baked beans and other pulses	99	87	96	116	101	98
Vegetables including all baked beans and other pulses	114	106	99	132	121	99
Fruit and vegetables, no fruit juice or baked beans/pulses	157	112	95	205	172	99
Fruit and vegetables (including one portion fruit juice, and/or one portion baked beans and other pulses)	174	133	96	228	193	99
Fruit and vegetables (including all fruit juice and all baked beans and other pulses)	200	154	99	277	234	99
Base = number of respondents			110			723

Note: * Composite dishes were for fruit: fruit pies, and for vegetables: vegetable dishes, including for example vegetable lasagne, cauliflower cheese and vegetable samosas.

Table A7(b)

Average daily amount (grams) of fruit and vegetables consumed by whether someone in respondent's household was receiving certain benefits: women consumers

Grams and percentages

Fruit and vegetables	Whether receiving benefits					
	Receiving benefits			Not receiving benefits		
	Mean	Median	% consumers	Mean	Median	% consumers
	g	g		g	g	
Excluding composite dishes:						
Fruit, no fruit juice	90	48	67	130	99	86
Fruit including one portion fruit juice	107	76	69	148	119	88
Fruit including all fruit juice	148	89	73	175	138	91
Vegetables, no baked beans/pulses	73	63	92	108	99	99
Vegetables including one portion baked beans and other pulses	75	65	92	109	99	99
Vegetables including all baked beans and other pulses	85	77	95	120	110	99
Fruit and vegetables, no fruit juice or baked beans/pulses	135	97	95	219	185	99
Fruit and vegetables (including one portion fruit juice, and/or one portion baked beans and other pulses)	152	111	95	239	208	100
Fruit and vegetables (including all fruit juice and all baked beans and other pulses)	195	140	97	278	236	100
Including composite dishes*:						
Fruit, no fruit juice	90	48	68	130	99	87
Fruit including one portion fruit juice	107	74	71	148	118	88
Fruit including all fruit juice	146	86	74	175	138	91
Vegetables, no baked beans/pulses	78	69	94	115	104	99
Vegetables including one portion baked beans and other pulses	80	70	94	116	106	99
Vegetables including all baked beans and other pulses	89	83	97	128	118	99
Fruit and vegetables, no fruit juice or baked beans/pulses	140	103	96	228	194	100
Fruit and vegetables (including one portion fruit juice, and/or one portion baked beans and other pulses)	157	116	96	248	220	100
Fruit and vegetables (including all fruit juice and all baked beans and other pulses)	200	147	97	286	244	100
Base = number of respondents			150			741

Note   * Composite dishes were for fruit: fruit pies, and for vegetables: vegetable dishes, including for example vegetable lasagne, cauliflower cheese and vegetable samosas.

Table A8

Average daily amount (grams) of fruit and vegetables consumed: consumers and all respondents

Grams and percentages

Fruit and vegetables	Consumers			All including non-consumers	
	Mean	Median	% consumers	Mean	sd
	g	g		g	g
Excluding composite dishes:					
Fruit, no fruit juice	120	87	79	95	109
Fruit including one portion fruit juice	139	108	81	113	120
Fruit including all fruit juice	169	128	84	143	150
Vegetables, no baked beans/ pulses	103	90	98	101	69
Vegetables including one portion baked beans and other pulses	106	93	98	103	70
Vegetables including all baked beans and other pulses	119	108	99	118	73
Fruit and vegetables, no fruit juice or baked beans/pulses	199	161	98	196	149
Fruit and vegetables (including one portion fruit juice, and/or one portion baked beans and other pulses	220	182	99	217	158
Fruit and vegetables (including all fruit juice and all baked beans and other pulses)	262	220	99	260	184
Including composite dishes*:					
Fruit, no fruit juice	120	87	81	96	110
Fruit including one portion fruit juice	138	108	82	114	120
Fruit including all fruit juice	169	129	85	144	150
Vegetables, no baked beans/ pulses	109	96	98	107	72
Vegetables including one portion baked beans and other pulses	112	99	98	110	72
Vegetables including all baked beans and other pulses	125	114	99	124	75
Fruit and vegetables, no fruit juice or baked beans/pulses	206	169	99	203	152
Fruit and vegetables (including one portion fruit juice, and/or one portion baked beans and other pulses)	227	189	99	225	161
Fruit and vegetables (including all fruit juice and all baked beans and other pulses)	270	226	99	268	187
Base = number of respondents			*1724*		

Note: * Composite dishes were for fruit: fruit pies, and for vegetables: vegetable dishes, including for example vegetable lasagne, cauliflower cheese and vegetable samosas.

Appendix B   Sampling errors and statistical methods

1   Sampling errors

This section examines the sources of error associated with survey estimates and presents sampling errors of survey estimates, referred to as standard errors, and design factors for a number of key variables shown in this volume. It should be noted that tables showing standard errors in the main part of this volume have assumed a simple random sample design. In testing for the significance of the differences between two survey estimates, proportions or means, the standard error calculated as for a simple random sample design was multiplied by an assumed, conservative, design factor of 1.5 to allow for the complex sample design.

The estimates presented in the main part of this volume are based on data weighted to correct for differential sampling probability and for differential non-response. The sampling errors presented in this appendix were calculated after applying a weight to compensate for differential sampling probability and differential non-response. The sample was also post-stratified, so that it matched the population distribution in terms of age, sex and region[1].

1.1 The accuracy of survey results

Survey results are subject to various sources of error. The total error in a survey estimate is the difference between the estimate derived from the data collected and the true value for the population. It can be thought of as being comprised of random and systematic errors, and each of these two main types of error can be subdivided into error from a number of different sources.

1.1.1   Random error

Random error is the part of the total error which would be expected to average zero if a number of repeats of the same survey were carried out based on different samples from the same population.

An important component of random error is sampling error, which arises because the estimate is based on a survey rather than a census of the population. The results of this or any other survey would be expected to vary from the true population values. The amount of variation depends on both the size of the sample and the sample design.

Random error may also arise from other sources such as the respondent's interpretation of the questions. As with all surveys carried out by the Social Survey Division (SSD), considerable efforts were made on this survey to minimise these effects through interviewer training and through feasibility work; however, it is likely some effects will remain that are not possible to quantify.

1.1.2   Systematic error

Systematic error, or bias, applies to those sources of error that will not average to zero over a number of repeats of the survey. The category includes, for example, bias due to omission of certain parts of the population from the sampling frame, or bias due to interviewer or coder variation. A substantial effort is put into avoiding systematic errors but it is likely that some will remain.

Non-response bias is a systematic error that is of particular concern. It occurs if non-respondents to the survey, or to particular elements of the survey, differ significantly in some respect from respondents, so that the responding sample is not representative of the total population. Non-response can be minimised by training interviewers in how to deal with potential refusals and in strategies to minimise non-contacts. However, a certain level of non-response is inevitable in any voluntary survey. The resulting bias is, however, dependent not only on the absolute level of non-response, but on the extent to which non-respondents differ from respondents in terms of the measures that the survey aims to estimate.

Although respondents were encouraged to take part in all components of the survey, some refused certain components. The Response Chapter of the Technical Report[2] examines the characteristics of groups responding to the different parts of the survey package. The analysis of the region, sex and age profile of respondents compared with population estimates showed evidence of some response bias. In particular, there was an under representation of men and of people aged 19 to 24 years. The data for the main part of this volume (and all subsequent volumes) were therefore weighted for differential non-response by sex, age and region.

1.2   Standard errors for estimates for the NDNS of adults aged 19 to 64 years

As described in Chapter 1 and Appendix D of the Technical Report[2], this survey used a complex sample design, which involved both clustering and stratification. In considering the accuracy of estimates, standard errors calculated on the basis of a simple random sample design will be incorrect because of the complex sample design.

This dietary survey sample was clustered using postcode sectors as primary sampling units (PSUs). Clustering can increase standard errors if there is a lot of variation in characteristics between the PSUs, but little variation within them. By contrast, stratification tends to reduce standard errors especially where the stratification factors are correlated to the survey estimate. Stratifiying the sample ensures that certain sections of the population are represented in the

sample. The main stratifier used on this survey was Standard Statistical Region (SSR). The PSUs were further stratified by population density, socio-economic group and car ownership (see Appendix D of the Technical Report[2]).

In a complex sample design, the size of the standard error of any estimate depends on how the characteristic of interest is spread within and between PSUs and strata: this is taken into account by pairing up adjacent PSUs from the same strata. The squared differences in the estimates between successive PSUs from the same strata are calculated and summed to produce the standard error.

The majority of estimates in this survey take the form of ratio estimates, either means or proportions. The formula to calculate the standard error of these is:

$$se\ (r) = \frac{1}{x}\ [var(y) + r^2 var\ (x) - 2r\ cov(y,\ x)]^{1/2}$$

where the ratio $r = y/x$.

The method explicitly allows for the fact that the percentages and means are actually ratios of two survey estimates, both of which are subject to random error. The value se (r) is the estimate of the standard error of the ratio, r, expressed in terms of se(y) and se(x) which are the estimated standard errors of y and x, and cov(y, x) which is their estimated covariance. The resulting estimate is slightly biased and only valid if the denominator is not too variable[3]. The ratio means for age groups have standard errors equal to zero for the full sample, because both the numerator and the denominator have been set to equal the population totals and thus cannot vary for any selected sample.

The method of standard error estimation compares the successive differences between totals of the characteristic of interest for adjacent PSUs (postal sectors)[4]. The characteristic is the numerator (for example, the average number of portions of fruit and vegetables consumed daily), and the sample size is the denominator in the ratio estimate[5]. The ordering of PSUs reflects the ranking of postal sectors on the stratifiers used in the sample design.

Tables B1 and B2 give standard errors, taking account of the complex sample design used on this survey, for the key variables presented in this volume. Standard errors for estimates of socio-demographic subgroups, such as household benefit status and region, are shown separately for men and women to reflect the way they are presented in the main part of the report. Standard errors are presented for the responding sample and the diary sample.

1.3 Estimating standard errors for other survey estimates

Although standard errors can be calculated readily by computer, there are practical problems in presenting a large number of survey estimates. One solution is to calculate standard errors for selected variables and, from these, identify design factors appropriate for the specific survey design and for different types of survey variable. The standard error of other survey measures can then be estimated using an appropriate design factor, together with the sampling error assuming a simple random sample.

1.3.1 The Design Factor (deft)

The effect of a complex sample design can be quantified by comparing the observed variability in the sample with the expected variability had the survey used a simple random sample. The most commonly used statistic is the design factor (*deft*), which is calculated as a ratio of the standard error for a survey estimate allowing for the full complexity of the sample design (including weighting), to the standard error assuming that the result has come from a simple random sample. The *deft* can be used as a multiplier to the standard error based on a simple random sample, $se(p)_{srs}$, to give the standard error of the complex design, $se(p)$, by using the following formula:

$$se(p) = deft \times se(p)_{srs}$$

Tables B1 and B2 show *deft* values for certain measures for all respondents and for those who completed a seven-day dietary record. The level of *deft* varies between survey variables, reflecting the degree to which the characteristic is clustered within PSUs or is distributed between strata. Variables that are highly correlated to the post-strata should also have reduced *deft* values. For a single variable, the level of the *deft* can also vary according to the size of the subgroup on which the estimate is based because smaller subgroups can be less affected by clustering.

Table B1 shows the *deft* values for a range of socio-demographic variables for the responding sample; and analogous variables in Table B2 for the diary sample. Table B2 also gives the *deft* value for the main analytic variable for fruit and

vegetable intake. For the socio-demographic variables, where geographic clustering would be expected, in both tables, six out of ten of the design factors for men and eight out of ten for women are less than 1.2. Design factors of this order are considered to be small and they indicate that, in this survey, the characteristic is not markedly clustered geographically. For two of the ten socio-demographic variables *deft* values are above 1.5 for both sexes. The *deft* value for the average daily number of portions of fruit and vegetables, including composite dishes and one portion of fruit juice and/or baked beans and other pulses, consumed is less than 1.2 for both men and women.

(Tables B1 and B2)

1.3.2 Testing differences between means and proportions

Standard errors can be used to test whether an observed difference between two proportions or means in the sample is likely to be entirely due to sampling error. An estimate for the standard error of a difference between percentages assuming a simple random sample is:

$$se_1(p_1-p_2)=\sqrt{[(p_1q_1/n_1)+(p_2q_2/n_2)]}$$

where p_1 and p_2 are the observed percentages for the two subsamples, q_1 and q_2 are respectively ($100-p_1$) and ($100-p_2$), and n_1 and n_2 are the subsample sizes.

The equivalent formula for the standard error of the difference between the means for subsamples 1 and 2 is:

$$se_2(diff) = \sqrt{(se_1^2+se_2^2)}$$

Allowance for the complex sample design is then made by multiplying the standard errors se_1 and se_2 from the above formula by their appropriate *deft* values.

In this volume the calculation of the difference between proportions and means assumed a *deft* value of 1.5 across all survey estimates. The calculation of complex sampling errors and design factors for key characteristics show that this was a conservative estimate for some characteristics for some age and sex groups, but was an optimistic estimate for other characteristics. Therefore there will be some differences in sample proportions and means that are not commented on in the text, but that are significantly different, at least at the $p<0.05$ level. Equally, there will be some differences that are described as significant in the text, but that are not significantly different when the complex sampling design is taken into account. An indication of the characteristics for which significance tests are likely to provide false-positives or false-negatives can be gained by looking at the size of the *deft* values in the tables in this appendix.

Confidence intervals can be calculated around a survey estimate using the standard error for that estimate. For example, the 95% confidence interval is calculated as 1.96 times the standard error on either side of the estimated proportion or mean value. At the 95% confidence level, over many repeats of the survey under the same conditions, 95% of these confidence intervals would contain the population estimate. However, when assessing the results of a survey, it is usual to assume that there is only a 5% chance that the true population value will fall outside the 95% confidence interval calculated for the survey estimate.

References and endnotes

[1] Weighting for different sampling probabilities results in larger sampling errors than for an equal-probability sample without weights. However, using population totals to control for differential non-response tends to lead to a reduction in the errors. The method used to calculate the sampling errors identifies the weighting for unequal sampling probabilities and to the population separately, and adjusts the sampling errors accordingly.

[2] The Technical Report, including its Appendices, is available online at: http//www.food.gov.uk/science/ (last verified November 2002).

[3] This variability of the denominator can be measured by the coefficient of variation of x, denoted by $cv(x)$, which is the standard error of x expressed as a proportion of x:

$$cv(x) = \frac{se(x)}{x}$$

It has been suggested that the ratio estimator should not be used if $cv(x)$ is greater than 0.2. For the standard errors produced here, the denominators for the ratios were 'number of men' and 'number of women'. Both of these totals were constant, determined by the post-stratification and, therefore, there is no variation in these denominators and hence the cv of the denominator will be zero.

[4] The calculation of standard errors and design factors for this survey used the software package Stata. For further details of the method of calculation *see*: Elliot D (1999). A comparison of software for producing sampling errors on social surveys. *Survey Methodology Bulletin* 44, pp 27–36. January 1999.

[5] For a survey of this kind, the sample size is subject to random fluctuation, both within each PSU and overall. This is because the number of adults identified in each PSU is dependent on which households are sampled and there will be differing amounts of non-response. There is more control in the (weighted) sample sizes of subgroups such as age and sex since these variables were used as post-stratifiers.

Table **B1**

True standard errors and design factors for socio-demographic characteristics of the responding sample by sex of respondent

Responding sample   Numbers

	Men			Women		
	% (p)	Standard error of p*	Design factor	% (p)	Standard error of p*	Design factor
Age group						
19–24 years	13	0.00	0.00	12	0.00	0.00
25–34 years	26	0.00	0.00	24	0.00	0.00
35–49 years	30	0.00	0.00	36	0.00	0.00
50–64 years	30	0.00	0.00	29	0.00	0.00
Region						
Scotland	9	0.90	1.06	8	0.83	1.03
Northern	28	1.04	0.76	25	0.87	0.68
Central, South West England and Wales	34	2.29	1.60	37	2.17	1.54
London and the South East	29	2.22	1.61	30	2.17	1.61
Household receipt of benefits						
Receiving benefits	14	1.29	1.24	18	1.33	1.17
Not receiving benefits	86	1.29	1.24	82	1.33	1.17
Sample size		1088			1163	

Note: * The ratio means for age groups for the responding sample have standard errors equal to zero because both the numerator and the denominator have been set to equal the population totals and thus cannot vary for any selected sample.

Table **B2**

True standard errors and design factors for socio-demographic characteristics of the diary sample and average daily intake of fruit and vegetables, including composite dishes, by sex of respondent: fruit and vegetables (all fruit juice counted as one portion; all baked beans and other pulses counted as one portion)

Diary sample   Numbers

	Men			Women		
	% (p)	Standard error of p	Design factor	% (p)	Standard error of p	Design factor
Age group						
19-24 years	12	0.85	0.75	11	0.70	0.68
25-34 years	25	1.01	0.67	24	0.79	0.56
35-49 years	31	0.78	0.49	36	0.81	0.50
50-64 years	32	0.94	0.58	29	0.78	0.51
Region						
Scotland	8	0.89	0.97	7	0.84	0.99
Northern	27	1.37	0.89	24	1.23	0.86
Central and South West England and Wales	36	2.65	1.59	38	2.79	1.72
London and South East	29	2.45	1.55	31	2.64	1.71
Household receipt of benefits						
Receiving benefits	13	1.46	1.24	17	1.46	1.17
Not receiving benefits	87	1.46	1.24	83	1.46	1.17
	Mean r	Standard error of r	Design factor	Mean r	Standard error of r	Design factor
Fruit and vegetables (all fruit juice counted as one per portion; all baked beans and other pulses counted as one per portion)	2.77	0.07	1.04	2.90	0.07	1.10
Sample size		833			891	

Appendix C   Unweighted base numbers

Table C1

Unweighted base numbers: dietary interview and seven-day dietary record by sex of respondent

Numbers

	Dietary interview	Seven-day weighed intake dietary record
Age		
Men aged (years):		
19–24	86	61
25–34	219	160
35–49	394	303
50–64	309	242
All men	1008	766
Women aged (years):		
19–24	109	78
25–34	277	211
35–49	487	379
50–64	370	290
All women	1243	958
Region		
Men		
Scotland	80	53
Northern	267	195
Central, South West and Wales	337	274
London and the South East	324	244
Women		
Scotland	111	70
Northern	341	256
Central, South West and Wales	436	350
London and the South East	355	282
Household receipt of benefits*		
Men		
Receiving benefits	145	106
Not receiving benefits	863	660
Women		
Receiving benefits	283	199
Not receiving benefits	960	759
All	**2251**	**1724**

Note: * Receipt of benefits was asked of the respondent about themselves, their partner or anyone else in the household. Benefits asked about were Working Families Tax Credit, Income Support and (Income-related) Job Seeker's Allowance.

Appendix D   Glossary of abbreviations, terms and survey definitions

Benefits (receiving)	Receipt of Working Families Tax Credit by the respondent or anyone in their household at the time of the interview, or receipt of Income Support, or (Income-related) Job Seeker's Allowance by the respondent or anyone in their household in the 14 days prior to the date of interview.
COMA	The Committee on Medical Aspects of Food and Nutrition Policy.
CAPI	Computer-assisted personal interviewing.
CASI	Computer-assisted self-interviewing. The respondent is given the opportunity to enter their responses directly on to a laptop computer. This technique is used to collect data of a sensitive or personal nature, for example, contraception.
Cum %	Cumulative percentage (of a distribution).
DH	The Department of Health.
Diary sample	Respondents for whom a seven-day dietary record was obtained.
dna	Does not apply.
GHS	The General Household Survey: a continuous, multi-purpose household survey, carried out by the Social Survey Division of ONS on behalf of a number of government departments.
HNR	Medical Research Council Human Nutrition Research, Cambridge.
Household	The standard definition used in most surveys carried out by the Social Survey Division, ONS, and comparable with the 1991 Census definition of a household was used in this survey. A household is defined as a single person or group of people who have the accommodation as their only or main residence and who either share one main meal a day or share the living accommodation. *See* McCrossan E. *A handbook for interviewers*. HMSO (London,1991).
HRP	Household Reference Person. This is the member of the household in whose name the accommodation is owned or rented, or is otherwise responsible for the accommodation. In households with a *sole* householder, that person is the household reference person; in households with *joint* householders, the person with the *highest* income is taken as the household reference person – if both householders have exactly the same income, the *older* is taken as

the household reference person. This differs from Head of Household in that female householders with the highest income are now taken as the HRP and, in the case of joint householders, income then age (rather than sex then age) is used to define the HRP.

lc	low calorie.
MAFF	The Ministry of Agriculture, Fisheries and Food.
Mean	The average value.
Median	*see* Percentiles.
MRC	The Medical Research Council.
na	Not available, not applicable.
NDNS	The National Diet and Nutrition Survey.
nlc	Not low calorie.
No.	Number (of cases).
ONS	Office for National Statistics.
PAF	Postcode Address File: the sampling frame for the survey.
Percentiles	The percentiles of a distribution divide it into equal parts. The median of a distribution divides it into two equal parts, such that half the cases in the distribution fall (or have a value) above the median, and the other half fall (or have a value) below the median.
Portion	A portion of fruit or vegetables is equivalent to 80g consumed weight.
PSU	Primary Sampling Unit: for this survey, postcode sectors.
Region	Based on the 'Standard regions' and grouped as follows:

Scotland

Northern
North
Yorkshire and Humberside
North West

Central, South West and Wales
East Midlands
West Midlands
East Anglia
South West
Wales

London and the South East
London
South East

The regions of England are as constituted after local government reorganisation on 1 April 1974.

	The regions as defined in terms of counties are listed in Chapter 2 of the Technical Report, online at: http://www.food.gov.uk/science/ (last verified November 2002).
Responding sample	Respondents who completed the dietary interview and may/may not have co-operated with other components of the survey.
SD/Std Dev	Standard deviation. An index of variability that is calculated as the square root of the variance, and is expressed in the same units used to calculate the mean (*see* mean).
se	Standard error. An indication of the reliability of an estimate of a population parameter, which is calculated by dividing the standard deviation of the estimate by the square root of the sample size (*see also* SD/Std Dev).
SSD	The Social Survey Division of the Office for National Statistics.
Wave; Fieldwork wave	The three-month period in which fieldwork was carried out.

Wave 1: July to September 2000
Wave 2: October to December 2000
Wave 3: January to March 2001
Wave 4: April to June 2001

| WHO | World Health Organization. |

Appendix E   List of tables

Appendix A: Fruit and vegetables

Tables

Appendix B: Sampling errors and statistical methods

Tables

B1   True standard errors and design factors for socio-demographic characteristics of the responding sample by sex of respondent

B2   True standard errors and design factors for socio-demographic characteristics of the diary sample and average daily intake of fruit and vegetables, including composite dishes, by sex of respondent: fruit and vegetables (all fruit juices counted as one portion; all baked beans and other pulses counted as one portion)

Appendix C: Unweighted base numbers

Tables

C1   Unweighted base numbers: dietary interview and seven-day dietary record by sex of respondent

Printed in the United Kingdom by The Stationery Office
ID 120071 C7 11/02 790695 19585

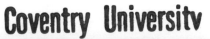